THE CHANGING SHAPE OF NURSING PRACTICE

The role of nurses in the hospital division of labour

Davina Allen

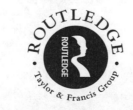

London and New York

First published 2001
by Routledge
11 New Fetter Lane, London EC4P 4EE

Simultaneously published in the USA and Canada
by Routledge
29 West 35th Street, New York, NY 10001

© 2001 Davina Allen

Typeset in 10/12pt Times by
The Midlands Book Typesetting Company Ltd
Printed in Great Britain by
St Edmundsbury Press, Bury St Edmunds, Suffolk

British Library Cataloguing in Publication Data
A catalogue record for this book is available
from the British Library

Library of Congress Cataloging in Publication Data
A catalog record for this book has been requested

ISBN 0-415-21648-6 (hbk)
ISBN 0-415-21649-4 (pbk)

CONTENTS

ACKNOWLEDGEMENTS

This book is based on my PhD research. Thanks are due:

To the staff of Woodlands Hospital, I am deeply grateful to them for their friendliness and for their candour in sharing with me their social worlds.

To my supervisors, Veronica James and Robert Dingwall, for their constructive criticism and for forcing me to ask difficult questions. I owe them an enormous intellectual debt.

To David Hughes for giving me opportunities after graduation that laid important foundations for this work and for his continuing encouragement and friendship.

To Alan Aldridge, Michael King and the late Annie Oakley, for saying the right things at the right time. Without them none of this would ever have happened.

To my partner, Richie, for his unwavering encouragement and support and invaluable technical guidance.

To my children, Sam, Megan and Susie, for understanding beyond their years, and to Mum and Tanya, for always being there.

To Alison Pilnick, Lesley Griffiths, Christina Luke, Ben Hannigan, Morag Prowse and Patricia Lyne who have been so much more than colleagues.

To Patricia Lyne, Morag Prowse and Carl May for their helpful comments on earlier drafts of the manuscript and also Robert Dingwall, who has been particularly generous with his time and advice.

To Christine Greenow for administrative support.

The writing of the book was greatly facilitated by a sabbatical from the Nursing, Health and Social Care Research Centre, School of Nursing and Midwifery Studies, University of Wales College of Medicine, Cardiff. The original project was funded by a Department of Health Nursing and Therapists Research Training Studentship. My thanks to Elizabeth Scott and her colleagues in the Research and Development

Division. The opinions expressed herein are my own and do not represent those of the Department of Health.

This book employs material which has appeared in a different form elsewhere. Chapters 5 and 7 draw on Allen, D. (2000) 'Doing occupational demarcation: the 'boundary-work' of nurse managers in a District General Hospital', *Journal of Contemporary Ethnography* 29(3):326–356, by permission of Sage Publications, Inc. Chapter 6 draws on Allen, D. (1998) 'Record-keeping and routine nursing practice: The view from the wards', *Journal of Advanced Nursing* 27: 1223–30, by permission of Blackwell Science, Ltd, UK. Chapter 7 draws on Allen, D. (1997) 'The nursing–medical boundary: a negotiated order?', *Sociology of Health and Illness* 19(4): 498–520, by permission of Blackwell Publishers and Allen, D. and Lyne, P. (1997) 'Nurses' flexible working practices: some ethnographic insights into clinical effectiveness', *Clinical Effectiveness in Nursing,* 1(3): 131–40 by permission of the publisher Churchill Livingstone. Chapter 8 uses material from Allen, D. (2000) "'I'll tell you what suits me best if you don't mind me saying", 'Lay participation in health care', *Nursing Inquiry,* in press Blackwell Science Ltd, UK.

ABBREVIATIONS

BP   Blood pressure
CMT   Clinical Management Team
CNA   Chief Nurse Advisor
DH   Department of Health
DHSS   Department of Health and Social Security
DNS   Director of Nursing Services
DTI   Department of Trade and Industry
ECG   Electrocardiograph
EN   Enrolled Nurse
GMC   General Medical Council
GNC   General Nursing Council
HCA   Health Care Assistant
HO   House Officer
IV   Intra-venous
IVI   Intra-venous infusion
NHS   National Health Service
NHSME   National Health Service Management Executive
NVQ   National Vocational Qualification
RCN   Royal College of Nursing
RN   Registered Nurse
SHO   Senior House Officer
TPR   Temperature, pulse and respirations
UGM   Unit General Manager
UKCC   United Kingdom Central Council for Nursing, Midwifery and Health Visiting

TRANSCRIPTION
CONVENTIONS

Tape-recorded interview material appears in italics.
Indented extracts in normal font indicate fieldnotes unless otherwise stated.
All tape-recorded materials and documents are verbatim transcriptions.
[...] words, phrases or sentences of the extract omitted.
[descriptive material added by the researcher in order to make the context and/or meaning clear]
Data have been edited in order to preserve anonymity.
All names of people and places are pseudonyms.

INTRODUCTION

This book is about the changing shape of nursing work in the hospital setting. 'Shape' is employed in the title in a literal sense to refer to the content of nurses' work, but it may also be read metaphorically, as an allusion to the state or status of nursing as an occupation. The work of hospital nurses can be understood as 'changing' in two respects: first, in relation to the place nursing occupies within the overall societal division of labour and, second, in terms of the routine fluctuation of work boundaries that individual practitioners experience in their daily working lives. Both may affect, and are affected by, nursing's occupational status in the wider society. The extent to which change is occurring in this latter respect is less certain.

These linked themes are examined herein through the analysis of five key nursing boundaries: nurse–nurse, nurse–support worker[1], nurse–management, nurse–doctor and nurse–patient. Based on ethnographic research undertaken on a medical and a surgical ward in a large UK district general hospital, the data reflect the experiences of most patients and staff. The study was carried out at a critical point in UK nursing's occupational development, when changes in health policy (DH 1989a) and in nursing and medical education (DHSS 1987; UKCC 1987; GMC 1993) had created considerable uncertainty as to the future shape of the nursing role. These policy changes provided a natural laboratory for a study of the division of labour because it is in such conditions of uncertainty and flux that the social and political processes through which occupations are formed are thrown into sharp relief (Strauss 1978: 105–41).

The policy developments that framed the research are examined in Chapter 1. Central to this was Project 2000 (UKCC 1987) and the advent of the 'new public management' (Hood 1991) in health care (DH 1989a). I argue that these developments rekindled deep-rooted historical tensions between 'professional' and 'service' versions of nursing, generating considerable ambiguity and confusion as to the legitimate nursing role. At the time of the research, debates about the future shape of nursing work reverberated throughout the occupation and health policy circles. The sorts of questions that were being raised in this context included: In what ways should nurses be developing the scope of their practice? Should they be undertaking doctor-devolved activities or colonizing new task areas? What should the role of the support worker be? Who should perform hands-on care? My aim, in undertaking the study, was to explore the ways in which nurses at the point of service delivery were managing the boundaries of their work and producing nursing in the light of these renewed debates about its occupational niche.

Throughout this book the boundaries of nursing work are taken to be a practical accomplishment. Although much intellectual energy is often expended in establishing the 'essence' of nursing, I adopt the line that the shape of nursing practice is, at root, the product of the locally situated actions and interactions in which nurses engage in the course of their everyday activities. Whether it be in the corridors of the Royal College of Nursing or the Department of Health, in lecture theatres in schools of nursing, on the wards or in the local accident and emergency department, nursing jurisdiction is 'done'. However, these social processes do not take place in a vacuum. To paraphrase Marx's famous dictum, people make history but not in circumstances of their own choosing. The accomplishment of nursing jurisdiction is fashioned in important ways by broader constraints – key examples are gender and economic stringency – and also by local factors such as members' practical concerns and the demands of the work setting. Although the effects of the former may be felt in common, there is much greater variation in the local features of the diverse environments in which nurses work. The corollary of this is that nursing jurisdiction is highly situated, that is, the way that it is 'done' varies in different locales. This conceptualization of nursing work has its theoretical origins in sociological theories of the division of labour and feminist scholarship, which are examined in Chapter 2.

Chapter 3 introduces the study setting and describes the research. Understanding the processes through which a study was executed is important in order that the reader can assess the validity of the findings. Moreover, as research and development becomes an increasingly stable fixture in the nursing world, it is my hope that this piece will stand as a useful example of how the ethnographic method can be employed in the study of nursing and give some flavour of what doing research of this kind is like (for other recent examples see, Wolf 1988; Anspach 1993; Porter 1995; Savage 1995). Reading Johnson's (1975) and Wax's (1971) accounts of doing research were an invaluable part of my own fieldwork preparations. For these reasons the methodological detail is probably lengthier than is usual in monographs of this kind. Nevertheless, the version that appears here has been considerably distilled from the original, and readers with a particular interest in the research process are referred to the full account in the thesis (Allen 1996).

When this study was originally conceived it was my intention to examine the nurse–doctor and nurse–support worker interfaces, as these were the divisions of labour that were the focus of the policy debates taking place at the time. Nevertheless, I was also clear that I wanted to examine the boundaries of nursing practice which were defined as important *by nurses themselves*. To this end I employed the concept of 'dirty work' (Hughes' 1984) as an initial sensitizing device.

In pointing to the presence of dirty work, Hughes was drawing attention to differences in the degree of honour and prestige associated with different kinds of work. In many of his empirical studies Hughes was concerned with work defined as 'dirty' by the dominant value system of a society, particularly the consequences of doing dirty work for members' sense of self. Indeed, it is in this sense that the concept has traditionally been employed in the analysis of nursing work (see, for example, Hendry and Martinez 1991; Lawler 1991; Somjee 1991). Yet dirty work may also be a reflection of a particular occupational perspective. Hughes argues that insofar as every occupation carries with it a self-conception, a notion of personal dignity, then it is likely that some of the work that its members do may threaten this dignity. This idea has been taken-up and developed by Emerson and Pollner (1976) in their examination of the origins of mental health workers' designation of certain tasks as 'shit work'. In this study staff considered their role to be the provision of psychotherapeutic work, and yet their everyday responsibilities involved them in crisis intervention scenarios where they operated as agents of social control. Emerson and Pollner argue that the designation of work of this kind as 'shit work' enabled staff to distance themselves from those activities they found threatened their occupational identity and, in so doing, mark the boundaries of their practice.

> Just as [...] embarrassment shows that the actor is aware of and committed to the moral order that his (sic) particular act has just violated, so the designation of dirty work reaffirms the legitimacy of the occupational moral order that has been blemished.
> (Emerson and Pollner 1976: 244)

It was in this sense that I felt the concept of dirty work could be used in the study of nursing in order to identify work that was symbolically polluting from the perspective of clinicians themselves. In practice this meant approaching the research setting with a sensitivity to those aspects of their work nurses attempted to distance themselves from or complained about. By attending to the ways in which they talked about their work, it became evident that, in addition to the medical and support worker interfaces, there were other boundaries that were of equal importance to nurses in their everyday practice: nursing's intra-occupational division of labour, the boundary between ward-based nurses and management and the boundary between nurses and patients.[2] The research focus was therefore modified to accommodate these emergent themes.

The first of these divisions of labour is explored in Chapter 4 in which I describe ward nurses' attempts to implement 'new nursing' (Salvage 1988) models of practice and analyse the implications that this had for the intra-occupational allocation of work. I argue that both wards were marked by tensions between senior nurses and the rest of the nursing team and that these appeared to stem from the contradictions and ambiguities in the professional and management discourses with which they were expected to grapple.

In Chapter 5 I focus on the nurse–support worker boundary and explore the processes through which it was being produced in a number of arenas in the study site. I analyse the demarcatory practices nurse managers employed in taking role realignment forward in the management arena and contrast this state of affairs with the situation on the wards where fuzzy work boundaries were the norm.

Chapter 6 examines the relationship between ward-staff and nurse managers. I trace the effects of the new managerialism at ward level and explore the 'named nurse' initiative and the nursing record as examples of how an apparent congruence between professional and management discourses can have a devastating impact on the shape of nursing work in the real world of hospital practice. In the second part of the chapter attention is turned to the nurse managers. I describe the considerable discomfiture they felt in taking forward many of the initiatives with which they were charged and explain how they accommodated themselves to these tensions by taking control of policy developments as they arose and deploying them for professional purposes.

Chapter 7 focuses on the nurse–doctor boundary. It begins with an exploration of the negotiations that took place between nursing and medical managers in implementing role realignment and the boundary disputes to which this gave rise. This picture of contested boundaries in the management arena is contrasted with the ward situation where, as with the nurse–support worker boundary, grass-roots staff were accomplishing shifts in the division of labour with little evidence of overt conflict.

In Chapter 8, I examine the nurse–patient boundary in the context of recent attempts within nursing and health policy to refashion the relationship between professionals and the lay public. I argue that although the allocation of tasks between nurses and patients was changing in the study site, modifications to their role relationship were less evident and traditional power imbalances remained intact. I argue that current understanding of this key caring interface has been hamstrung by a paucity of theorizing in this area and suggest that the conceptual framework developed in this book offers a potentially useful starting point for taking forward further empirical work.

In Chapter 9 I attempt a synthesis of the five boundaries examined in the book and consider the implications of recent developments in nursing and health policy for the future shape of nursing practice.

The text may be read at a number of levels: for its substantive content, that is, as an exploration of the processes through which an important area of the hospital division of labour is routinely worked out in everyday practice; for its analytic and theoretical content, that is, as a new way of thinking about the nursing role; as an illustration of the application of sociological theories to nursing work; and as an example of ethnography as a method for researching nursing practice.

1

PROFESSIONALISM AND MANAGERIALISM

Project 2000 will bring out highly-trained professionals who we will have to use properly [...] Nurses are locking themselves in too tight a definition. What's a doctor and what's a nurse? There's work to be done, you get the work done by the people who are best qualified to do it [...] Hands-on care is below nurses' level of competence. The nurse will become the overall assessor of the care that the individual needs to have [...] A higher quality, cheaper service, with a competitive edge will be achieved by those who make the most improvement in their labour costs. It's just common sense.

(Eric Caines[1] in an interview with Naish 1990, quoted by Naish 1993: 25)

It may appear that many nursing activities can be performed by untrained people ... Nurses use (bathing, washing and other forms of personal care) ... to perform other vital activities. Bathing is an ideal opportunity for observation of the skin and pressure areas. Counselling, reassurance and health education are carried out in a variety of settings when patients are relaxed and feel able to talk. Replacing trained nurses with untrained ones wherever possible will save money in the short term, but will prevent trained nurses having the vital and regular informal contact with patients and will affect the quality of total holistic care that nurses strive to deliver.

(Rosemary Gillespie, letter to the *Guardian,* 15 May 1993, quoted in Davies 1995: 89)

These extracts were precipitated by developments that were taking place in the UK in the 1990s in which changes in health policy (DH 1989a) and medical and nursing education (DHSS 1987; UKCC 1987; GMC

1993) had created vigorous debates about the future shape of the nursing role. They suggest very different versions of nursing and are assembled in rhetorically distinctive ways. Caines uses the language of management with its emphasis on quality, economy, efficiency, and competition. Gillespie employs a professional discourse that stresses the importance of holistic care and the value of combining physical tending with counselling, reassurance and health education. Both are oriented to a 'common sense' understanding of nursing work. Caines makes an appeal to the (self-evident) mundaneness of hands-on care, whereas Gillespie aims to counter 'what everybody knows' by making visible the indeterminacy and complexity of nursing practice.

The interaction of the discourses of professionalism and managerialism has had a major historical influence on the definition of nursing as an occupation and on the evolution of its jurisdiction. At the end of the nineteenth century, for example, Nightingale's vocational vision of nursing as a 'moral métier' (Rafferty 1996) vied with the professional model advocated by Mrs Bedford Fenwick founded on scientific skills. The struggle over nurse registration centred on the very different visions of nursing they proposed and was infused with the politics of gender and economic interest.

Nightingale advocated a 'domestic academy' model of nurse training in which the education of nurses was principally about the formation of 'character'. Rafferty (1996) argues that the roots of this approach can be found in Victorian ideas about the role of middle-class women as guardians of morality in the home. Improving the morals of nurses was seen as a route to the reform of the working class. The Bedford-Fenwick group, committed to a professional version of nursing, adopted a strategy that emphasized technical and scientific skills based on the model of the medical profession. While not denying the importance of character, Mrs Bedford-Fenwick insisted that the good nurse was both technically competent and morally virtuous.

At the end of the nineteenth century, nursing was tightly linked to particular hospitals and the knowledge nurses gained was not readily transferable to other types of patient or institutional context. Nightingale's conception of nursing as a calling akin to a religion, coupled with a strategy of on-the-job training, provided hospitals with a cheap, disciplined and compliant labour force (Witz 1992). The registrationists were anxious to break the monopolistic control of the hospitals over the career prospects of nurses. Mrs Bedford-Fenwick proposed a private-practice model of nursing, based on a generalizable training that would prepare nurses to work with a wide range of patients in and outside the hospital. The absence of a national scheme of accreditation meant that the voluntary hospitals enjoyed a series of captive labour markets. Mrs Bedford-Fenwick's proposal threatened to remove this control and place it in the hands of an autonomous professional body; instead of nurses working on terms set by the hospitals, the hospitals would have to employ nurses on terms set by the occupation (Dingwall *et al*. 1988).

Opposition to nurse registration was expressed in gendered terms. Emphasis was given to the importance of the training institution in instilling an appropriate character in nurses so that they did not abuse their intimate relationship with patients. Books and theory could be no guarantee of virtue it was argued. This anti-intellectualism was further underwritten by arguments that stressed nurses' uneducatability and that derived a gloss of scientific legitimacy from evolutionary biology. Rafferty (1996) cites the example of Dyce Duckworth's address to the Scottish Society of Literature and Art in which he cautioned against higher education for women lest it should disrupt 'the natural evolution of perfect womanhood' (p. 59).

In the event, the 1919 Nurses Registration Act proved to be a hollow victory for Mrs Bedford-Fenwick's professional vision. As Dingwall *et al*. (1988) and Rafferty (1996) have argued, it appeared to have been influenced by the government's intention to create a national health service after the war that would require some rationalization of nurse training, rather than sympathy for the registrationist case. The Act established a register of trained nurses and a General Nursing Council (GNC) charged with its maintenance and the determination of conditions. The Bedford-Fenwick group fought within the GNC for a system based on the model followed by the medical profession in which standards for recruitment and training were independent of the staffing needs of the hospital (Rafferty 1996). They were a minority voice, however, and in the early years of the Council priority was given to the development of a wider dispersion of skills and to the encouragement of local arrangements to rationalize training provision (Dingwall *et al*. 1988). Moreover, although the Registration Act gave nurses a protected title – only nurses on the register could call themselves state registered – this was not a prerequisite for employment as a nurse and, as a consequence, despite their desire for an all-qualified work force, faced with recurrent recruitment crises, the professionalizers were unable to resist the introduction of the EN (enrolled nurse)[2] in 1943 and the unplanned growth of the nursing auxiliary.

Nursing work is now a long way removed from its Victorian origins, yet this historical legacy remains centrally relevant to our understanding of the shape of the occupation today. While given a contemporary flavour, the struggle between the discourses of professionalism and managerialism is as germane as we begin the twenty-first century as it was at the end of the nineteenth. In the UK in the 1990s, the implementation of Project 2000 and the introduction of general management into the National Health Service (NHS) resulted in a revival of these divergent visions of nursing jurisdiction, marking a critical point in the occupation's development.

Nursing and the new managerialism

In the late 1980s and early 1990s, the UK, like other countries in the developed and developing world, witnessed major reforms of its health care system. Signalling the start of a period of profound change in the nature of public administration, 'new public management' (Hood 1991) in the NHS began with the publication of the Griffiths Report (DHSS 1983) and was further consolidated in the 1990 NHS and Community Care Act. This 'management revolution' (Klein 1995) was part of a systematic attempt to refashion the relationship between public sector professionals and the state by exercising greater control over their practice and use of resources. It was the medical profession that was the principal target of the government's agenda for change in the health sector, but the reforms that they instituted also had important implications for the shape of nursing work.

At the time, these were arguably the most radical policies instigated by any administration, but concern with NHS governance was by no means new. The search for improved management has been a persistent feature of the NHS's evolution (Harrison *et al.* 1990), reflecting two linked tensions that arise from its organizational form. The first is the relationship between central government and local provision and the difficulties of reconciling central funding and accountability with the need for sufficient autonomy to meet local needs (Ranade 1994). The second is the product of an historical bargain struck between the state and the medical profession at the NHS's inception (Klein 1995), which accorded doctors a privileged place in administering the new system (Ranade 1994). Although government controlled the budget, doctors controlled what happened within the budget. This was a double-edged arrangement for both parties. On the one hand, operating within tightening financial constraints, the medical profession was left to do the government's dirty work in rationing service provision. On the other hand, the considerable clinical autonomy doctors enjoyed meant less central control over how resources were utilized. Klein (1995) describes this as a truce rather than a final settlement and, from the 1960s onwards, these strains became increasingly apparent.

These linked tensions constitute the so-called NHS management 'problem', which has been the basis of successive reforms of the service. Interest in improved management gathered momentum in the late 1960s and early 1970s, reflecting rising concern with the alleged poor performance of the 'government machine' (Harrison *et al.* 1990) and changing management ideologies in relation to the whole of the public sector (Flynn 1990). Previously, service organizations had been seen as unique but this was replaced by the belief that they were equally amenable to the principles of economic rationality associated with business organizations. Planning was seen as a neutral tool. Targets could be set and progress made towards them (Allsop 1984). The emphasis on achieving greater efficiency and rationality through planning was common to both main political parties (Klein 1995) and these ideas were manifest in a number of health policies throughout the 1960s and 1970s.

By the end of this period, however, there was mounting concern over the NHS. Spiralling costs and a series of industrial disputes led to the questioning of existing health policies. The 1979 Conservative government, in strong contrast to its 1970s predecessor, was not committed to the ideology of rational planning (Klein 1995). In the reorganization it instituted in 1982, decision making was devolved to local level although interestingly, they did not propose any fundamental reform of management. Indeed, ministers were emphatic that this was to remain firmly in health professionals' hands. Launching *Patients First* Patrick Jenkin, then Secretary of State for Social Services, argued:

> I believe that doctors and other professional people in the NHS are trained to take professional decisions off their own bat, and do not need the torrent of advice to which in recent years they have been subjected. It is doctors, dentists and nurses and their colleagues in the other health professions who provide the care and cure of patients, and promote the health of the people. It is the purpose of management to support them in giving that service.
>
> (Allsop 1984: 139, quoting DHSS and Welsh Office 1979)

This was a view that was to be short-lived.

The publication of the Griffiths Report in 1983 marked a clear turning point in NHS management policy. In the past, the main preoccupation had been with the structure of the NHS; attention now shifted to its organizational dynamics (Klein 1995). *Griffiths* proposed major changes to NHS organization, duties, responsibilities, accountability and control. A general management structure from top to bottom was prescribed (Dingwall *et al.* 1988) with a number of in-built mechanisms to ensure accountability to central government. Although the introduction of general managers was, to a considerable extent, a mechanism for changing doctors by bringing them into the managerial process and instilling managerial values, it had a devastating effect on nursing. Nurses already had a management structure, and since the 1974 reorganization had been directly responsible for the enormous budgets that covered the provision of nursing staff (Davies 1995). '[A]t a stroke', however, 'the 1984 reorganization removed nursing from nursing's own control and placed it firmly under the new general managers' (Strong and Robinson 1990: 5).

Griffiths challenged many of the assumptions that had shaped the NHS since its inception. Consumerism emerged as a key theme in response to the criticism that services were oriented to the needs of providers rather than its users.

> The NPM [new public management] claims to speak on behalf of taxpayers and consumers and against cosy cultures of professional self-regulation. Taxpayers and citizens, rather like shareholders, are the mythical reference points that give the NPM its whole purpose.
>
> (Power 1999: 44)

The rhetoric of this period cast the general public as knowledgeable consumers of health services and emphasis was given to information and issues of communication. The period saw a dramatic increase in the number of complaints about health services provision and the implementation of local systems for measuring user satisfaction. Working at the 'front-line' of service delivery, it was frequently nurses who found themselves at the sharp-end of this new consumer consciousness (Annandale 1996).

The reforms were underpinned by a very particular view of 'management' (Flynn 1990). Many of the changes were introduced by people from the private sector and the managerialist ethic that developed was grounded in the belief that managers should 'manage', that they should be in control of their organizations and be proactive. 'Active' management was to replace 'passive' administration. The demand for greater 'value for money' generated a raft of techniques for management evaluation and control of clinical activity (Elston 1991) and signalled the beginning of an era in which the provision of care became subject to continuous scrutiny. In the NHS, as in other areas of public service provision, audit and accounting practices assumed a decisive function (Power 1999).

In addition to encouraging health professions to embrace a more 'business-like' approach, the new managerialism was also underpinned by a belief that it was possible to manipulate organizational cultures in a more direct way (Ouchi 1981; Deal and Kennedy 1982; Peters and Waterman 1982; Schein 1985). Commonly referred to as the 'corporate culture' paradigm, exponents of this view claim that 'excellence' is dependent on organizational members sharing common values and goals (Hughes and Allen 1993a). Although many NHS managers did not embrace these ideas uncritically, their influence was nevertheless evident in the discourse they adopted (Pettigrew *et al.* 1988; Traynor 1999). Pettigrew *et al.* (1988), for example, write of the spread into NHS management of a new language of 'product champions', 'visionaries' and 'change agents' (Hughes and Allen 1993a).

But *Griffiths* was only a beginning. In 1990, as a consequence of increasing concern with cost containment, the health service was reorganized again. The reforms introduced as a result of the National Health Service and Community Care Act 1990 were in many ways a logical development and strengthening of the *Griffiths* management philosophy, but their 'kernel' – the creation of the quasi-market – was a radical new departure (Ranade 1994). The crucial components of the Act were:

- the creation of a split between purchasers and providers of health care;
- the institution of a contracting process whereby providers would present tenders to purchasers;
- the creation of 'self-governing Trusts' that, following the Conservative victory at the General Election in April 1992, became the normal means for the provision of secondary and community health care; and
- other related policies, such as budgets held directly by general practitioners for certain services.

(Paton 1993)

Consonant with the consumerist trend was the introduction of the *Patient's Charter*, one of a series of citizen's charters that aimed to 'improve and modernize the whole range of public services and to set standards that the general public can expect and demand' (Robertson 1994: 86, quoted by Lyne 1998). Standards were specified in relation to matters such as waiting times for outpatient appointments and surgery (Hughes and Griffiths 1999). Aggregate data was used as the basis for 'league tables' by which Trusts' 'performance' could be assessed. Health Authority contracts for clinical services often included 'penalty clauses' which resulted in reduced payment to Trusts that failed to meet the targets set (Hughes and Griffiths 1999; Griffiths and Hughes 2000).

One way in which *Griffiths* had tried to control doctors was by bringing them under the sphere of influence of general managers. When this brought only limited success, the reverse tactic of involving doctors in management was attempted through the 'Resource Management Initiative' (Packwood *et al.* 1991). The 1991 reforms entailed the extension and acceleration of these trends. A key feature was the formation of a system of clinical directorates, in which medical, nursing and management staff worked together to manage speciality budgets. These devolved freedoms were coupled with much tighter systems of accountability.

The reforms also entailed an emphasis on human resource management. This was another area of considerable devolution. In the past there had been a heavy reliance on centralized national negotiations of terms and conditions of employment, with local activity being mainly concerned with hiring and firing and dealing with individual grievances. In the context of market competition, however, the ability to manage one's own work force could be of paramount importance (Paton 1993). The reforms gave Trusts the autonomy to set the pay and conditions of service of their work force and decide upon the size and skill-mix of their staff (Robinson 1994). Although the rhetoric linked local pay to performance, initially individual and then later Trusts, in the nursing context certainly, these developments had rather more to do with the ability to restructure jobs and respond to local market conditions (Harrison and Bruscini 1995). 'Skill-mix' and 'reprofiling' became vogue phrases, raising fundamental issues about the demarcation of work responsibilities (Paton 1993).

> As part of this initiative, local managers, in consultation with their professional colleagues, will be expected to re-examine all areas of work to identify the most cost effective use of professional skills. This may involve a reappraisal of traditional patterns and practices.
>
> (DH 1989a: 15)

In an important parallel development, the White Paper: *Opening New Markets: New Policy on Restrictive Trade Practices* (DTI 1989) paved the way for staff to be employed on the basis of competencies (Shaw 1993). Non-professional staff could now be employed to carry out those tasks traditionally reserved for those with the professional qualification, providing competence could be demonstrated (Brown 1990; cited by Shaw 1993).

Of crucial importance for nursing were parallel developments in medical education (DHSS 1987; GMC 1993) and the initiative to reduce the hours worked by junior hospital doctors. The *New Deal* (NHSME 1991) set firm limits on junior doctors' contracted hours (72 per week or less in most hospital posts) and working hours (56 hours per week). Local task forces were established throughout the UK and given the power to recommend the removal of education approval from a training post if the standards had not been achieved. The *New Deal* called for an increase in the number of career grade (non-training) posts and encouraged new ways of organizing junior doctors' work such as shifts, partial shifts and cross-cover between specialities. It also suggested the 'sharing' of key clinical tasks by nurses and midwives, providing the impetus for a range of initiatives throughout the UK that shifted the boundary between medical and nursing work (see, for example, Allen and Hughes 1993; Allen *et al.* 1993; Hughes and Allen 1993b).

At the time of the fieldwork, the reforms had been in place 4 years. In practice there had been less competition between providers in the NHS than had been anticipated. Most purchasers and providers were locked into permanent relationships and hence 'purchasers' became 'commissioners'. Furthermore, the internal market had become the managed market: a recognition that purchasing was about shaping the services available to a local population in the long term as opposed to buying off-the-shelf to satisfy immediate wants (Klein 1995). Moreover, although the rhetoric was about autonomy, diversity and devolution (Allsop 1995), the managed market turned out to be one in which politicians were active actors (Klein 1995).

A number of commentators have underlined the immense difficulties of assessing the impact of the reforms (Robinson and Le Grand 1994; Allsop 1995; Klein 1995). Klein (1995) argues that because the reforms marked the beginning of a process of experiment and adaptation it was impossible to come to any firm conclusions as to where things were going or what had been achieved. Furthermore, there was little official interest in evaluating their effects. Indeed, as Pollitt (1995) observes, it is a fundamental irony of the new public management that its insistence on the importance of measurable outputs in health care has not, in turn, been applied to itself. Notwithstanding these considerations, however, there are some points about which more certain conclusions can be drawn. First, the reforms conspicuously failed to achieve the objective as set out in *Working For Patients*, of giving patients 'greater choice of services available' (Allsop 1995; Klein 1995). On the contrary, regional disparity in services meant that an individual's access to health care could hinge to a considerable extent on their postcode. Second, little progress was made towards the government's general aim of bringing about increased satisfaction and rewards for those working in the NHS (Klein 1995). Third, although the reforms successfully challenged the inherited patterns of work in the NHS, their effects were most acutely felt by professions allied to medicine: inroads into the power of the medical profession have been limited (Ham 1992; Dent 1993; Harrison and Pollitt 1994; Exworthy 1998). Increased participation of doctors in hospital management represents not so much the subordination of clinicians to managers as the emergence of clinician managers.

At the time of writing, the UK health care system is undergoing yet further change. The internal market has been abolished and collaboration and partnership are to replace competition as the primary drivers of service provision. Policy rhetoric has shifted from a preoccupation with consumers and efficiency to concern with quality and equity. The implications of these developments for nursing will be considered in Chapter 9. I now want to examine the other shaper of nursing practice: the discourse of professionalism.

Nursing and the new professionalism

Project 2000 (UKCC 1987) was the UKCC's[3] proposal for the reform of nursing structure, practice and pre-registration education. An explicit professionalizing strategy, it was an attempt to uncouple the historical ties between nurse education and health service provision, and an ambitious plan to create a practitioner-based division of labour (Davies 1995). Its proponents believed that it had the potential to overcome some of the occupation's most persistent problems: low status, poor retention, and the lack of a clearly defined area of expertise underpinned by a scientific body of knowledge (Beardshaw and Robinson 1990).

The Project 2000 reforms were wide-ranging, radically altering a system of training that had been criticized for many years. Although there was a growing number of university-based degree programmes, prior to the first pilot schemes for the reforms 98 per cent of nurse education took place within schools of nursing (RCN 1985, cited by Meerabeau 1998), which were managed by Directors of Nurse Education who were generally accountable to the District Health Authority. Student nurses, who were employees of the District Health Authority, underwent a separate training according to their chosen speciality. This lasted 2 years for ENs and 3 for RNs (registered nurses). During this time learners constituted a significant element of the hospital labour force.

Project 2000 established a single point of entry to nurse training by abolishing the EN grade of nurse; existing ENs were offered the possibility of undertaking conversion courses leading to RN status. Nurse education was relocated to institutes of higher education. All non-degree nurses were to follow an 18-month common foundation programme followed by 'branch' programmes for particular specialities – adult, child, mental health and learning disability. Learners' contribution to service provision was reduced from 60 to 20 per cent. There was a shift to a health, rather than a disease-oriented, curriculum, an emphasis on people in the wider socio-cultural context and practical placements that aimed to prepare students for work in a range of institutional and non-institutional settings. Academic skills were to be valued and rewarded by a Diploma in higher education.

Project 2000 was founded on a particular philosophy that had profound implications for nursing culture and practice. 'New nursing' (Salvage 1988), as it has come to be known, began in the UK in the early 1970s with departments of nursing in universities and polytechnics generating an interest in nursing theory (Salvage 1992). Academic nurses drew heavily on the work of American nurse theorists who were seeking to define nursing's unique contribution to health care in order to establish a domain of autonomous practice and epistemological demarcation from medicine. At the time, an important means to this end was the nursing process.

The idea that nursing was a process rather than a separate set of activities was first introduced by Hall in 1955. The concept emerged at a point when widespread structural changes within American society and medicine coincided with increasing disaffection within nursing with its occupational status and the quality of patient care (Salvage 1992; De la Cuesta 1983). Initially employed as an educational tool, the nursing process has also been described as a form of documentation, a method of organizing nursing work and a professionalizing philosophy.

In the UK, the nursing process first began to be discussed during 1973 but no articles were published on the subject until 1975. Once arrived, diffusion and institutionalization were rapid (Aldridge 1994). By 1977 it was being implemented at hospital level. The period prior to its emergence was one of considerable discontent and debate. British nurses were seeking satisfactory methods of working and there were a number of precursors to the nursing process that prepared the ground for its dissemination: patient-centred care, patient assignment, total patient care, team nursing, and progressive patient care (De la Cuesta 1983). Walton (1986) suggests that the greatest catalyst for its implementation came in 1977 when, in revising its general nursing syllabus, the GNC exhorted schools of nursing to use the nursing process to 'provide a unifying thread for the study of patient care and a helpful framework for nursing practice' (GNC 1977; quoted by Walton 1986: 1).

'New nursing' ideology had important implications for the organization of nursing work. It was a welcome reaffirmation of the clinical, as opposed to the administrative, skills of nurses. In the past, the practice of staffing hospital wards with a combination of qualified nurses, auxiliaries and learners at different stages of training, had resulted in the development of a system of work based on hierarchical task-allocation (Melia 1987; Proctor 1989). As a number of authors have pointed out, the management discourse that dominated nursing for a large part of its occupational development led to the distinction made by Goddard (1953) between 'basic' and 'technical' nursing care becoming overlaid with a skills hierarchy (McFarlane 1976; Melia 1979). Under this method of work organization nurses moved from one patient to another carrying out tasks that were allocated to them according to their place in the ward status system. Increasing seniority meant less 'hands-on' contact with patients. 'New nursing' promised to reverse these trends and replace this fragmented system of care delivery with a holistic approach in which the performance of tasks was integrated into the total care of the patient. The patient is seen as a whole person for whom all aspects of healing work are essential. In this vision of nursing, 'basic' tasks such as bathing are given a central place in the qualified nurse's work, and accorded equal importance as supposedly, more scientific or technical tasks handed down to nurses from doctors (Salvage 1992).

'New nursing' theorists advocate primary nursing as the system of work organization that supports these aspirations for practice. Primary nursing involves allocating 24-hour responsibility for each patient to a trained nurse, who plans, gives, supervises and evaluates care, wherever possible with the active collaboration of the patient and his or her family. The primary nurse leads a team of other nurses – known as associate nurses – who deliver care when the primary nurse cannot. Associate nurses administer the prescribed care. They do not take diagnostic or prescriptive decisions on their own behalf.

Until relatively recently, nursing jurisdiction was limited to care of the biological functioning of the patient (Armstrong 1983). 'New nursing' changed all this. In rejecting task-allocation it brought about a redefinition of the nursing role. Central to Hall's thought was the notion of therapeutic communication: nurses were instructed to engage with the patient as a subjective being. Exponents of 'new nursing' maintain that nursing is a therapy in its own right and that by the 'therapeutic use of self' (Travelbee 1966: 18; cited by Ersser 1997) nurses can help people to feel better and also get better (see, for example, Pearson 1988). The nurse–patient relationship is formulated as an equal partnership and it is through the establishment of a 'healing association' that nurses are said to promote healing. In more recent years these trends have taken a more spiritual turn. Drawing their inspiration from phenomenology, a number of nurse academics have underlined the function of nurses in assisting patients to find 'meaning' in their experiences. Indeed, according to some nurse theorists, health *is* expanding consciousness (see, for example, Newman 1986).

This reconstruction of the nurse–patient relationship has not been accepted uncritically. It is by no means clear, for example, if patients or nurses want the type of relationship held up by 'new nursing' as the ideal. As Salvage (1992) has pointed out, the immediate concern of patients is likely to be relief from pain and discomfort, rather than a meaningful relationship in which they can discuss their problems. Moreover, the part played by faith or belief might make an asymmetrical relationship beneficial (Salvage 1992) and management of the intimate activities that nurses sometimes undertake for patients may actually be facilitated by a more detached approach (see, for example, Lawler 1991; Savage 1995). In a rare empirical study of nursing's therapeutic effects, Ersser (1997) found that nurses and patients seldom referred to the 'therapeutic use of self'. He writes:

> The informants made limited reference to the importance of the nurses' actions being intentional and deliberative, with, for example, evidence of emotional labour. In contrast they gave many indications of the therapeutic importance of the nurses' 'everyday' or 'ordinary social interaction' which are not of an intentional nature, such as the nurses' friendliness and impact on the ward atmosphere.
>
> (Ersser 1997: 296)

Indeed, the lack of research into the ways in which patients respond to this new approach to their care has been used to support the claim that the reconstruction of the nurse–patient relationship has been driven more by the desire to solve nurses' problems of occupational legitimacy rather than by the needs of patients (Dingwall *et al.* 1988).

To note some of the difficulties with Project 2000 and its associated ideologies is not to undermine the importance of its aspirations for practice but to highlight the fact that the movement must also be understood

13

as a specific professionalizing strategy that aims to enhance the status and rewards of the occupation. As Traynor points out:

> Nurses have generally been more comfortable understanding themselves as working on a project of liberation from oppression than acknowledging themselves as implicated in the very same power moves as those who they see as oppressing them. Many nurses are able to critique effectively the medical institution as engaged in a process of maintaining a significant power base, marshalling biomedical knowledge as one of its resources, but they appear to often take at face value the nursing profession's own rhetoric of holism, patient advocacy, professionalism or feminism, unwilling to understand those arguments and rhetorics as cultural resources, discourses that are adopted to further the profession's desire for power.
>
> (Traynor 1999: 63)

Because Project 2000 conflated the attempt to improve nursing education and practice with the pursuit of functional autonomy it was flawed by a profound insensitivity to the reality of nursing work. For example, the characteristic emphasis of 'new nursing' ideology on a close interpersonal relationship between patient and nurse is at odds with the reality of much hospital nursing where nurses work with multiple patient assignments that have to be co-ordinated with the needs of a complex organization. Moreover, primary nursing is predicated on the assumption of a work force numerically dominated by qualified nurses but this is clearly contrary to the accumulative body of historical evidence (Dingwall *et al.* 1988) and dismissive of the economic realities of modern health care. In addition, as Porter (1992) has observed, the construction of nursing as an autonomous profession, independent of, and separated from, medicine bears little resemblance to the daily practice of most nurses.

On both sides of the Atlantic, studies continue to highlight the gap between nursing theories and nursing practice (Buckenham and McGrath 1983; De la Cuesta 1983; Melia 1987). Failure is frequently attributed to the education and preparation of practitioners but, as a number of authors have pointed out, these disappointments may be more accurately explained by the refusal of the proponents of 'new nursing' to take account of the fundamental nature of nursing work in a complex organization such as the modern hospital (De la Cuesta 1983; Milne 1985; Melia 1987; Keyzer 1988).

Historical antecedents

In the UK, the contemporary resurgence of professional discourses of nursing has its origins in the restructuring of the occupation that followed the Salmon Report (Ministry of Health 1966). This is a period of nursing's development that has been examined in depth by Carpenter (1977, 1978). Carpenter observes that for much of its early development nursing was characterized by two paradoxical features: an extraordinarily flexible jurisdiction and an extremely conservative infra-structure (Carpenter 1977; Davies 1977; Dingwall *et al.* 1988). On the one hand, the occupation willingly embraced a broad range of work activities brought together under the notion of the 'sanitary idea'. On the other hand, this was coupled with the insistence that nursing should be a life-long vocation that necessitated the continuation of a cloistered life and an authoritarian regime entailing the repetition of routine tasks (Carpenter 1977).

Carpenter (1977) argues that by the 1960s there had been phenomenal changes in nurses' job content. As a result of the growth of medical science, a number of clinical responsibilities had been delegated. There had also been an increase in the importance of the nurse as a co-ordinator of a range of ancillary functions. Nursing work was further affected by a rise in the numbers of chronically ill patients requiring long-term care. According to Carpenter (1977), the particular balance of forces at the beginning of the 1960s meant that it was the managerial, rather than the clinical, changes to nursing jurisdiction which were given emphasis.

As we have seen, the 1960s and 1970s were characterized by a general belief in the efficacy of management techniques in the public sector. Claims for managerial roles and equality of status with administrators became the strategy by which the health professions other than medicine sought to advance themselves (Harrison *et al.* 1990). As the largest single group of employees in the health service, nurses were an obvious target in the unrelenting drive towards rationalization. The Salmon reforms aimed to modernize nursing management to fit the new environments of the planned district general hospitals and achieve a more efficient use of labour (Dingwall *et al.* 1988). *Salmon* implemented a management structure that gave nursing parity with other interests in the NHS (Dingwall *et al.* 1988). The management chain was extended above and below the level of matron. The most significant change, however, was the progressive dilution of nursing by lower level staff. Armed with new strategies for disciplining the profession, the nursing elite abandoned their insistence on the centrality of routine duties to the occupation and redefined them as low status skills that could be delegated to support workers in the search for cost containment.

Carpenter points out that although the nursing elite maintained the pretence that in pursuing a strategy of control outside of the clinical sphere they were attempting to uplift the profession as whole, in actuality the gains of *Salmon* were very narrow. Equality of nursing with other groups in management was won by virtue of the elite's domination over the nursing labour force, an equality that posed little threat to the dominance of medicine in the clinical sphere. This led to considerable disillusionment with *Salmon* at the lower levels of the nursing hierarchy. The new managers were often seen as career-oriented with little interest in the practical situation. Moreover, the reforms created a formal structure that failed to reward clinical expertise: prestige and remuneration increased with distance from the bedside. The nursing elite had hoped the reforms would improve staff morale but the increased union and professional tensions between clinicians and managers that followed indicate that, in this sense certainly, *Salmon* was a spectacular failure.

Against this background of industrial unrest, the Briggs Committee was set up to review nursing education. Although given a contemporary flavour, the recommendations of the Briggs report (DHSS 1972) had clear resonances with the aspirations of Mrs Bedford-Fenwick: a nursing curriculum modelled on medical lines with a general foundation leading to specialist qualifications. Briggs advocated a 'comprehensive' vision of nursing education. This new training would encourage a mixed ability intake onto a common programme in which individuals would be able to choose a route and rate of learning that suited them. The curriculum would be modularized and its different elements could be repeated until mastered. The initial 18-month programme would lead to a Certificate. Registration would require a further 18 months of study and selected candidates would be able to continue to a Higher Certificate after that. Although graduate programmes were left outside of this structure, it was envisaged that they would be the main source of the future leaders of the profession. Briggs proposed a single powerful council to oversee the system with all the different sections of the occupation brought under its remit. It looked as if the professionalizers' ambitions were at last to be realized (Dingwall *et al.* 1988).

The publication of the bill in November 1978, however, was a bitter disappointment. It concentrated almost exclusively on the regulatory structure and gave virtually no attention to the educational questions that had been of such concern. At this time, the advocates of a professional version of nursing had their base mainly in the educational institutions. Dingwall *et al.* (1988) suggest that their response to Briggs was to use the classroom to promulgate their occupational ideals, and, as we have seen, a major mechanism for this was the nursing process.

The new professionalism and the new managerialism: tensions and convergence

It is clear, then, that the origins of Project 2000 are deeply rooted in nursing's occupational heritage. The removal of students from service provision, the creation of a core generic training, and the entry of nursing into higher education are the realization of many aspects of Mrs Bedford-Fenwick's 'professional' vision. Given that, in the past, elitist programmes of nursing reform have always been constrained by economic realities, why was Project 2000 different? There is a clue in the observation made by Rafferty (1992), that historically the success of nurse-driven policy changes can normally be traced to their synchronization with wider organizational and policy concerns. The 1919 Nurse Registration Act was a case in point.

One reason for the government's attraction to Project 2000 was the spectre of the 'demographic time bomb'. During the late 1980s policy-making was dominated by the unenviable prospect of having to recruit up to half of all the suitably qualified women school leavers in order to maintain NHS staffing and wastage levels. In this context, a small, highly skilled nursing core, supported by a pool of cheaper workers made for a more flexible work force that could be deployed to meet changing demographic and social trends (Carpenter 1993; Naish 1993).

There were also considerations of cost. A restructuring of nursing practice afforded the opportunity to make efficiency savings. Nursing salaries are one of the largest single items of public expenditure in the UK, consuming almost 3 per cent of the total (Dingwall *et al.* 1988). Government acceptance of Project 2000 entailed the important rider that nurses agree to a new training for support workers to be determined by the National Council for Vocational Qualifications (Beardshaw and Robinson 1990): a generic – non-nursing – accrediting body responsible for a wide range of work-based vocational and technical education. An important objective of the Project 2000 reforms had been to clearly differentiate qualified and unqualified staff, but the introduction of National Vocational Qualifications (NVQs) was likely to have precisely the opposite effect (Dingwall *et al.* 1988; Hughes 1993) by making alternative qualifications available at the level of, and in competition with, professional qualifications (Shaw 1993).

There is, moreover, a clear strain between the professional vision in which all aspects of nursing are carried out by qualified staff and that of management, which argues that this has to be set against the need to provide a cost-effective service. As Buchan (1992) observes, it was skill-mix alterations that the new health service managers concentrated on as the main source of cost savings, and soon after the implementation of Project 2000 there was evidence of dilution. Between September 1990 and 1991 the NHS lost 15,400 qualified nurses – a drop of 5.2 per cent – but the number of unqualified staff rose by 137,400, a rise of 17 per cent. This changed the ratio of qualified to unqualified staff from 61:23 to 58:28 (Ranade 1994: 32). As Dickson and Cole (1987) point out:

> [T]he ratio of helpers to nurses does not merely affect what the helper can and cannot do, but also what the nurse can and cannot do.
>
> (Dickson and Cole 1987: 25;
> quoted by Robinson *et al.* 1989: 1)

Paradoxically, this dilution of the nursing work force was occurring at exactly the same time as the drive to increase patient turnover, so that average acuity levels were actually higher.[4]

As Davies (1995) has shown, however, there was no explicit bargain struck at national level that nursing had to accept a restructuring in order to achieve educational change, and the question as to who should do what within the caring division of labour was never addressed. Rather, the onus was shifted to the Regional Health Authorities to produce individual plans for replacement staff and the number of entrants for admission to the new training programmes. Davies cites the work of Elkan *et al.* (1993), who paint a picture of *ad hoc* decisions, of choices sometimes being put in the ward sister's court as to whether she wanted more qualified staff, but too few of them to do the work, or more unqualified staff and a reversion to a task-oriented mode of work organization.

The creation of a more educated nursing work force also meant nurses would be better placed to take over doctor-devolved activities. In a parallel development, *The Scope of Professional Practice* (UKCC 1992) brought an end to the requirement that nurses needed medically sanctioned extended role certificates to undertake tasks not covered in basic training and shifted responsibility for managing the boundaries of nursing to individual practitioners themselves. Although the professional vision of nursing certainly supports role developments (see, for example, Sutton and Smith 1995) – for example, a number of nurses have integrated complementary therapies into their practice (Wright 1995) – the shape of nursing jurisdiction it envisages is not necessarily consonant with the management view, where considerations of cost, the desire for a flexible work force and the problem of junior doctors' hours figure prominently. Indeed, much of the impetus behind the 'new nursing' came from its leaders' desire to *differentiate* the nursing contribution from that of medicine.

A further attraction of the 'new nursing' from a management perspective is the amount of paperwork it generates. In the US, care plans became one of the accounting mechanisms by which planners endeavoured to curtail the escalating costs of medical care (Dingwall *et al.* 1988). In the UK, the nursing process has become an important tool for quality assurance programmes.

> There is a general consensus in the professions that providing patient care on an individualized basis, and developing and establishing monitoring and audit systems in each provider unit and in primary health care are the foundation stones of a high quality service, and that these elements should be included in the service contracts and will serve as bench marks in collaboration between purchasers and providers in their standards setting programme.
>
> (NHSME 1993: 10)

As we will see in Chapter 6, far from augmenting professional autonomy, the individualization of care, coupled with its detailed documentation, can actually increase the scope for external control over nursing, not by direct intervention but by standard setting (Dingwall *et al.* 1988; Salvage 1995). It also increases nurses' personal accountability for care delivery (De la Cuesta 1983; Salvage 1995) even though they may have little control over many of its constituent elements. Ironically, moreover, although 'new nursing' ideology brings nurse–patient relationships centre-stage, this kind of work is invisible to the language of business and is written out of the charts (Diamond 1988; Samarel 1991). Davies (1995) interprets these problems as a reflection of the masculine vision embedded in the new managerialism. She argues that the language of managerialism, with its targets and indicators, performance culture, rationality and gloss of scientific neutrality is blind to the business of caring.

The fragility of the consensus between 'new nursing' and the new managerialism finds its most explicit expression in the notion of the 'named nurse'. Standard 8 of *The Patients' Charter* states that every patient has the right to receive the care of a 'named nurse', midwife or health visitor. Although echoing the primary nursing ideal, these links were down-played in its implementation presumably because of the cost implications. Far from signifying government recognition of the value of nursing then, the 'named nurse' initiative might be more accurately understood as an attempt to appease a disillusioned electorate, a means of auditing service provision and a strategy for placing responsibility for quality care on individual nurses rather than on Trusts and government (Salvage 1995).

Rafferty (1996) notes that the convergence of government policy and the registrationist lobby in 1919 was more apparent than real. Similarly, new managerialism had the potential to undermine the professional vision of nursing in fundamental ways. This point is underscored by the failure of Project 2000 to achieve its principal aim: a demarcation between education and practice. In the event, the uncoupling of student service was accompanied by the attempt to establish a closer tying of supply and demand. As *Working For Patients: Education and Training; Working Paper 10* (DH 1989b) revealed, the ties of education to service was to be preserved through the mechanism of the internal market. Humphreys (1996; cited by Meerabeau 1998) argues that the government's primary concern was to ensure that educational costs did not contaminate the market principles of the NHS reforms. However, not only was the extension of the purchaser/provider model from service to education a long way from Project 2000's aim that programmes were education – not service – driven (Davies 1995), it had a devastating effect on the stability of nurse education.

Muddying the waters

In setting out the policy context that formed the background to this study, I have juxtaposed developments in health service management with the professional aspirations of nursing as embodied in the Project 2000 reforms. It is important, however, that the discourses of professionalism and managerialism should not be conflated with the distinction between nurses and managers. Historically, professional and management discourses can be found *within* nursing. Nursing is an extremely heterogeneous occupation (Carpenter 1977; White 1986; Melia 1987); the discourse of professionalism is not supported by all (Salvage 1985; Porter 1992) and a business culture may attenuate the clinical values of nurse managers (White 1986). Within the 'rank-and-file' it is possible to identify both professional and service views of the nursing role (McKee and Lessof 1992) and in nurses' everyday talk professional and management discourses are often intertwined (see, for example, Robinson *et al.* 1989; Traynor 1999).

Summary and conclusions

In this chapter I have examined the immediate policy context against which the study was carried out and have traced its historical antecedents. My exposition has been framed in terms of the tensions between professional and management discourses of nursing and their points of convergence and divergence. The revival of professional discourses of nursing in the 1990s, like the rise of management discourses in the 1960s, was the occupation's response to a crisis of legitimacy. These status anxieties were the product of wider social, organizational and technical changes that have wrought a similar crisis of legitimacy in health care more generally. The new public management was an attempt to develop a way forward following the break-down of the post-war consensus over the welfare state. These separate discourses project very different visions of the appropriate nursing role creating considerable jurisdictional ambiguity for practitioners. Both, however, are predicated on a platonic ideal of nursing work, which sociological analysis suggests is unwarranted. Far from being founded on some essentialist concept of nursing, in any given historical context the *actual* shape of nursing jurisdiction is the product of nurses' practical management of their work boundaries in the course of their everyday activities. The question of how nurses at the point of service delivery shaped the boundaries of their practice in the light of these renewed debates about the appropriate nursing role, was the starting point for this study.

2

CONCEPTUALIZING THE
NURSING ROLE

In this chapter I draw on sociological theories of the division of labour and the insights of feminist scholars to develop a non-essentialist conceptualization of the nursing role that is rooted in the work setting. My aim is to construct an analytic framework that can help us to understand the evolution of nursing as an occupation and its place within the division of labour in society, but which also provides the necessary theoretical tools to explicate the fine grain of workplace processes and the experiences of individual practitioners. In order to comprehend the dilemmas and contradictions of nursing work and to understand why nurses accomplish their work boundaries in the shape that they do, I wanted a perspective that recognized the volitional aspects of human action but was also cognisant of local, structural and historical constraints on agency. .

I begin with the work of Durkheim (1933) on the division of labour in society, and go on to explore the development of the major themes in his writings by Hughes (1984) and Abbott (1988). An overview of feminist insights into women and work follows. I suggest that, taken together, key elements of these theories provide a useful framework that can help us to understand nursing's occupational development and the value society accords to its work. In order to analyse the shape of nursing practice in the workplace, however, we also need to embrace theories that can handle the detail of social processes. To this end, the chapter concludes with an exploration of interactionist theories of the division of labour as developed in the writings of Freidson (1976, 1978) and Strauss and colleagues (Strauss *et al.* 1963, 1964, 1985; Strauss 1978). What follows is not intended to be a comprehensive review and critique of this body of work. Rather, it is an attempt to take what is useful in these perspectives and to combine them in a way that helps us to further understand the changing shape of nursing practice.

The division of labour as social ecology

My approach is predicated on two basic assumptions: that the world of work is analogous to an ecological system and that occupations are social phenomena. These were central themes in Durkheim's study, *The Division of Labour in Society* (1933, first published in 1893), and they have preoccupied sociologists ever since.

Durkheim

Durkheim observed that mechanization and the concentration of capital forces, brought about by the agrarian and industrial revolutions of the nineteenth century, had led to 'the extreme division of labour'. By this, he was referring to the occupational specialization of society as a whole and the separation of social life into different activities and institutions. It was the economic functions of the division of labour that had hitherto been given prominence in academic scholarship, but Durkheim was primarily concerned with its social significance. He believed that increased specialization in society generated mutual interdependence and thereby contributed to the maintenance of social integration. According to Durkheim, traditional types of society are characterized by 'mechanical' solidarity; their social cohesion is derived from likenesses and similarities. The growing complexity of society, he argued, had created a new basis of reciprocity arising from socio-economic specialization and an interdependence of parts; he called this 'organic' solidarity.

Durkheim points to the sexual division of labour as an example of work being divided on the basis of complementary differences. He claimed that as humankind has evolved, men and women have become increasingly different: women withdraw from public life and devote themselves to family and take care of 'psychic' functions while men perform the 'intellectual' ones. Durkheim saw this gendered division of labour in positive terms, but as feminist scholars have pointed out, the separation of social life into the public and the private has had long-lasting implications for women's lives and the value of the work that they do. Nursing is a prime example.

Durkheim believed that there is a continuing tendency for societies to move from mechanical towards organic solidarity. He proposes that 'if one takes away the various forms the division of labour assumes according to conditions of time and place, there remains the fact that it advances regularly in history' (Durkheim 1933: 233).[1] According to Durkheim, a highly specialized societal division of labour is caused by a rise in 'moral' and 'material' density. That is, there are increased numbers of people who are in sufficient contact to interact with one another. Durkheim also believed that occupational competition could accelerate the division of labour. Drawing on Darwin's ecological theories of natural selection, he argues that in a given society different occupations can coexist alongside one another in as much as they pursue different objectives, but the more alike their functions and the more points of contact they have, then the greater is the risk of conflict. Under conditions of conflict, he argues, occupations can disappear or transform, leading to a new specialization. As his critics (see, for example, Campbell 1981) have pointed out, however, Durkheim's emphasis on social integration led him to down-play the role of conflict in the world of work.

Hughes

As with Durkheim, central to Hughes' (1984) writings is the idea of the division of labour as a social system. Whereas Durkheim focused on its structure and function, Hughes places greater emphasis on its internal dynamics. Of central importance for Hughes are the peripheries and boundaries of occupations. For him, the division of labour was an unsatisfactory concept because it stresses divisions rather than connections between parts. He argues that it is impossible to describe the work of an individual without reference to that of others with whom they work.

Like Durkheim, Hughes also emphasizes the social significance of work but he considers it in more detail. He makes an analytic distinction between the role and task components of occupations. The 'technical division of labour' refers to the allocation of tasks ('what I do') and the 'moral division of labour' refers to one's role ('who I am'). Hughes maintains that the study of work should focus on the role people *think* they should practise in the workplace as well as the work they actually do. It is erroneous to try and study tasks separate from people, he argues.

As Freidson (1978) points out, Durkheim paid little attention to the concrete substance of the concept of the division of labour, whereas this is the focus of much of Hughes' attention. For Hughes, an occupation is comprised of a 'bundle' of tasks. Not all these tasks have the same value nor require the same types or degrees of skill. Both technical and role factors can affect the tasks in the bundle. They may be held together by the fact that they are performed by one person with a particular occupational title or because they seem natural parts of an occupational role. Alternatively, they may coalesce because they entail similar skills or because they can be conveniently carried out together. An activity within the bundle may be symbolically valued far beyond its importance, others may be considered 'dirty'. Hughes suggests that the history of an occupation can be described in terms of changes in these bundles of activity, and their value and function in the total system. For Hughes, the items of activity and social function that make up an occupation are historical products. The tasks in an occupational bundle are not fixed and their symbolic value may change as a result of other shifts in the system of work. Occupational mobility may involve the attempt to drop certain of these tasks and acquire others with higher symbolic value.

Studying American nursing in the 1950s, Hughes observed that with developments in medical technology, tasks were downgraded and delegated from the physician to the nurse, who passed other tasks down to the support worker. According to Hughes, the nurse was moving up nearer the doctor in technique and devoted more time to the supervision of other staff. New workers were coming in at the bottom to take over tasks abandoned by occupations ascending the mobility ladder. Hughes believed that the dropping of low prestige tasks was part of the process by which nursing was becoming a profession. As we saw in Chapter 1, nursing's current professionalizing strategy attempts to reverse these trends, reunifying previously devolved tasks (Brannon 1994). This underlines the importance of placing professional projects (Larson 1977) in their social and historical context (see, for example, Davies 1983).

Two key concepts in Hughes' thought are licence and mandate. Licence refers to the activities an occupation is granted to carry out by society, whereas mandate refers to the jurisdictional claims that are made by an occupation.[2] The scope of licence and mandate is not fixed: it can expand and contract. Any occupation may aspire to professional privileges by attempting to reconstruct its licence and expand its mandate. Some occupations have greater power to enlarge their licence and mandate than others. Professions, more than any other occupation, claim a broad licence and mandate. According to Hughes, occupations may try to gain a more secure standing by claiming professional status. They do this by a series of 'symbolic steps', for example, by increasing the educational qualifications required for entry to the occupation, by going into research, by asserting that themselves and not some outside authority shall judge what is their proper work, by putting their more routine duties onto the shoulders of others, and by claiming a mandate to define the public interest in matters relating to their work. Hughes suggests that by examining the ways in which occupations try to change themselves or their image, we can come to a greater understanding of what 'profession' means in our society.

Hughes was concerned with the commonalties of work. He insisted that the central problems of 'men (sic) at work' were the same and this appears to have led him to neglect consideration of the effects of gender on structuring the experience of work. For example, despite his interest in nurses' work and his insistence that any study would be meaningless unless developments on the boundaries of the occupation were taken into account, nowhere does he acknowledge that the division of labour between medicine and nursing is inherently gendered. Nevertheless, he was clearly sensitive to the consequences of gender for women and work. He taught his students how to understand the situation of women (Deegan 1995) and he recognized the possibility of gender segregation and sex-typing (Hughes 1984: 141–50). He also argued that '[a] woman may have a career in holding together a family or raising it to a new position' (Hughes 1984: 138). Although this sees women playing a limited role, it at least puts women's domestic work on a par with men's paid employment (Dex 1985). Nevertheless, it would seem that his interest in the development of concepts that would be widely applicable to the world of work and occupations led him to down-play the importance of gender.

Notwithstanding these criticisms, however, Hughes' contribution to the study of work is undoubtedly a valuable one. Although only loosely formulated, his ideas have been extremely influential, stimulating a wealth of empirical studies of work and the development of sociological theory. Abbott's (1988) *The System of Professions: An Essay on the Division of Expert Labour* is a recent example of the ways in which Hughes' ideas have been developed.

Abbott

Through a comparative historical study of the professions of nineteenth and twentieth century England, America and France, Abbott builds a detailed theory of professions. His chief concern is with the evolution and interrelations of professions, and how occupational groups control their skills and knowledge. According to Abbott, traditional theories of professionalization have been more concerned with the forms rather than the content of professional work. Case studies reveal that it is the content of the professions' work that is changing he argues. Abbott proposes that the proper unit of analysis should be the professional task area which he calls jurisdiction.

Jurisdiction is key to Abbott's thought. He uses the concept to develop Hughes' ideas on licence and mandate, although he is not himself explicit about this. According to Abbott, each profession is bound to a set of tasks by jurisdictional ties. Analysis of professional development is an analysis of how this link is created in work. For Abbott, jurisdiction has cultural and structural aspects. The cultural dimension of jurisdiction refers to the construction of tasks into professional problems. Professions are distinguished by the ways in which they control their knowledge and skill, he argues. Craft occupations emphasize control over technique *per se* but the distinguishing feature of professions is the centrality of abstract knowledge. Any occupation can obtain licensure or develop a code of ethics, but 'only a knowledge system governed by abstractions can redefine its problems and tasks, defend them from interlopers, and seize new problems [...] Abstraction enables survival in the competitive system of professions' (Abbott 1988: 9). As we saw in Chapter 1, nursing is engaged in precisely this kind of intellectual project.

Jurisdiction also has a social structure. Jurisdictional claims can be made in public, legal, and workplace arenas. In claims made in the public arena, it is assumed that there are clear boundaries between professions and that tasks can be objectively defined. Public images of jurisdiction typically last for decades. Formal control of work is conferred in the legal arena, however, and here jurisdictional claims are even more explicit. According to Abbott, the absolute necessity to abolish all uncertainty leads to an almost arbitrary definition of the margins of professional jurisdiction, and the boundary areas that are precisely delineated have little resemblance to real life situations.

The work setting is the third arena for jurisdictional claims that Abbott identifies. Here jurisdiction is the assertion of the right to control certain kinds of work. In open markets of independent practitioners, jurisdictional boundaries between competing professions are established by referral networks and similar structures. The situation is very different in an organization, however, where the division of labour often locates professionals in settings where they must assume umpteen extra-professional tasks and cede many professional ones. According to Abbott, formalized job descriptions are only loosely related to reality; the actual division of labour is established through negotiation and custom. He maintains that boundaries between professions in organizations can disappear, especially in overworked ones.

> There results a form of knowledge transfer that can be called workplace assimilation. Subordinate professionals, non-professionals, and members of related, equal professions learn on the job a craft version of a given profession's knowledge systems.
>
> (Abbott 1988: 65)

Abbott argues that this assimilation is encouraged by the fact that in a work situation it is the output of an individual not his or her credentialed status that is important. He underscores the profound contradiction between the formal arenas of jurisdictional claims – public and legal – and the informality of the workplace. According to Abbott, it is professionals who must accommodate this discrepancy.

Abbott argues that jurisdictional boundaries are perpetually in dispute, both in local practice and in national claims. 'It is the history of jurisdictional disputes that is the real, the determining history of the professions' (Abbott 1988: 2). The ultimate goal of most professions is full jurisdiction, argues Abbott, but given that professions constitute a system, there is a limit to the number of full jurisdictions to go round and so other kinds of settlement must be found. Occasionally, professions may share an area without an explicit division of labour; riot control is one such example. This has been claimed in the last 50 years by the military, by the police, by private police agencies and also social scientists. Another solution is for one profession to assume an advisory control over certain aspects of work. Medicine has expanded its jurisdiction by advancing advisory claims, argues Abbott. Professions may also divide their jurisdiction not according to the content of the work, but according to the client. There is some evidence of this kind of settlement at the medical–nursing interface in the case of nurse-practitioners who are providing services previously delivered by doctors but to very specific social groups – often those with polluted identities. An alternative settlement entails the subordination of one profession under another. Not only does this permit the superordinate profession to delegate routine work, it settles the complex legal and public relations between incumbent and subordinate from the start. This is essential given that subordination often involves extensive workplace assimilation and fuzzy occupational boundaries that would be a threat if public and legal jurisdiction were not already established. Abbott identifies the position of nursing in relation to medicine as an example of this latter form of jurisdictional settlement. This is a view that appears to be supported by social scientists and historians alike (Walby 1986; Dingwall et al. 1988; Gamarnikow 1991; Witz 1992; Davies 1995).

Abbott also examines the effects of the internal composition of individual professions on the overall system of work. According to Abbott, professions are internally differentiated and these differences both generate and absorb system disturbances. Abbott maintains that the most important division of labour is that which divides routine into non-routine elements, with the two falling to different segments of a profession or even to outside groups. According to Abbott, this results in the degradation of what was previously professional work to non-professional status.

This is sometimes accompanied by degradation of those who do that work. There is one exception to this rule, Abbott argues, and that is when the division of labour is tied to a career, as is the case in medicine. Recent developments in medical education in the UK suggest that this may now be changing as routine medical work is delegated to nurses and other health care workers.

In the final level of his analysis, Abbott examines the impact of wider social forces on the system of professions. He points to the technological and organizational changes of the nineteenth century that created vast areas of new work for professions and destroyed relatively few others. He also underlines the profound effects of changes in knowledge. According to Abbott, professions seek to legitimate their work by reference to the central value system of a given society and may thus be affected by changes in societal norms. He argues that the rising value of organizational efficiency and its concomitant emphasis on outputs has moved inter-professional competition away from conflict over social origins and general values towards conflict over measurable results. In the UK certainly, there is evidence of a further shift taking place that emphasizes public involvement and the integration of users, views into what were previously closed professional concerns.

The final facet of modern rationality that Abbott examines is the rise of the university. The presence of many professions on campus makes this another potential area for inter-professional competition – for example, over matters of funding and also questions as to who should teach what to whom. Nursing's relocation into higher education institutes has led to precisely these sorts of inter-professional conflicts as educators struggle to keep control over a nursing curriculum derived from an eclectic mixture of social and biological sciences. Having worked so hard to establish epistemological demarcation from medicine, recent developments in nursing academe may be understood as an attempt to safeguard nursing's control over its knowledge base in the face of competing claims from other disciplines such as the social sciences.

Abbott's thesis is detailed and wide-ranging, furnishing important conceptual tools that may be employed in the study of nursing. The model he proposes, however, is deficient on two counts. First, he gives insufficient weight to the importance of power in inter-professional competition. He assumes that no profession delivering bad services can stand indefinitely against competitors however powerful. If professions fail to deliver service he claims, then ultimately clients will go elsewhere. Even if this was empirically the case, it does not necessarily follow that power is therefore unimportant. For example, it ignores how dominant professions may control the ways of thinking about a problem and adjudicate success and failure. Furthermore, although Abbott acknowledges the importance of the central value system for professions' jurisdictional claims, he fails to acknowledge that the dominant societal ideas can systematically devalue the skills of certain groups within society, such as women, for example. Abbott maintains that he has chosen this model because he wishes to explain inter-professional conflict that others, using a power model, have treated as incidental and largely ignored. Arguably, however, acknowledgement of the importance of power within the theory would not necessarily close off the possibilities for explicating inter-professional conflicts. Indeed it might further our understanding of why they take the form that they do (see, for example, Witz 1992).

Second, although Abbott's systems approach is admirable, its restriction to professions is more problematic. He does not offer a definition of the term 'profession' and so we are left with the problem of identifying the boundaries of the system. Moreover, in ignoring work that falls outside 'the system of professions', Abbott excludes important areas from his analysis, for example, the relationship between work shared between a profession and, what Freidson (1978) has called, the 'informal economy'. Here Freidson is referring to legitimate economic activities that exist alongside the official work force, performed for money, goods or services. Among the full-time informal occupations the most conspicuous is the housewife. Historically the relationship between formal and informal caring has been crucial for nursing's professional project, both in terms of the value accorded to its work and also the career paths of its members. Furthermore, the boundary with family carers is assuming increasing salience for nurses and other paid carers. There is, then, a sense in which Abbott's thesis is both too systematizing and not systematizing enough. If the analytic focus is to be restricted to the system of professions then the limits of that system need to be more clearly specified. Given the problems in defining profession (Becker 1970; Roth 1974; Freidson 1983), however, arguably it is more fruitful to focus on the system of work as a whole, as do Hughes and Durkheim.

Although Durkheim, Hughes and Abbott pursue their analyses in different ways, certain commonalties emerge from their writing. Occupations are essentially social phenomena, that is, work has a meaning for those who do it. The division of labour is conceptualized as a social system. Social, economic, technological and organizational changes may impact upon the system of work and may reshape occupational boundaries. Changes within occupations also have ramifications for the wider system. New tasks may enter the system and others may leave or be passed on to other occupational groups. Emphasis is given to the connections and interrelations of the parts constituting the whole. The boundaries between different occupations expand, overlap and retreat in an ongoing evolutionary process. Durkheim emphasized structure and function, whereas Hughes and Abbott pay more attention to dynamism and process. In the combined insights of these authors we have the beginnings of a perspective that can be usefully employed in the analysis of nursing work. As I have indicated in my exposition, however, a third commonality in the perspectives reviewed thus far is the absence of critical attention to issues of gender.

Gender, work and nursing

For many years, issues of gender were largely ignored in sociological analyses of work. Not only was there a dearth of empirical accounts of women's work experiences, but many of the concepts employed in 'malestream' sociology have been based on inherently sexist assumptions (Dex 1985). As Stacey (1981) has pointed out, for a long time sociology persisted in dividing its subject matter into the two worlds of Adam Smith and Adam and Eve. On the one hand was the public world of work, class and industry and, on the other, was the private world of domestic life. One corollary of this was a tendency to equate 'work' with 'paid work outside the home', excluding women's unpaid work in the form of housework (Oakley 1974a,b) and motherhood (Oakley 1979). Furthermore, the relationship between the sexual division of labour in the domestic sphere and women's position in the public domain had been largely overlooked. More recently, however, a body of literature has emerged highlighting women's experiences and attempting to develop a satisfactory theoretical framework through which to understand their position in the world of work.

In the public sphere, work is divided by gender. The occupational structure is segregated by gender horizontally – with women and men working in different types of occupation – and vertically – with women concentrated in lower grade occupations (Hakim 1979). Nursing provides a powerful illustration of this point. More than 90 per cent of British nurses are women and yet men occupy a disproportionate share of senior posts (Davies 1995).

There is considerable debate as to the root causes of women's segregation in the occupational structure. Orthodox accounts have read women's position in the public sphere from their role in the private. It is suggested that women's patterns of work reflect the fact that their primary responsibilities are home-centred. But, as Needleman and

Nelson (1988) have pointed out, women's working patterns are often evidence of the lack of opportunity rather than the exercise of choice. Studies reveal that the work world is structured in a way that makes it extremely difficult for women to combine paid work and motherhood (Homans 1987). Work is organized as if every worker had a full-time housewife at home (Apter 1993). Moreover, the evidence suggests that irrespective of whether women work in the public sphere, responsibility for domestic work tends to rest squarely on their shoulders (Oakley 1974a; Hochschild 1990). The difficulties of combining paid work with domestic responsibilities and child-rearing means that women are particularly susceptible to exploitation by 'understanding' employers. They tend to be concentrated in part-time poorly paid work, which lacks employment protection, and have no training or paid holidays.

Davies (1995) has highlighted the failure of UK health service managers to rise to the challenge of managing a predominantly female work force. Historically the management of nursing labour has been based on a high recruitment/high waste model of womanpower in contrast to the low intake/low waste model of conventional manpower planning. Support for post-basic courses and continuing education is not treated in the same way as medicine because of the assumption that nurses will leave. Davies argues that a more woman-friendly approach to the management of the nursing workforce would work with a notion of lifetime participation and manage career breaks to enhance this. It would carry out cost-benefit studies of different forms of child-care that took into account the real costs of turnover and failures to return. It would look at flexible hours and consider reorganizing work schedules and individualizing hours.

Others have delineated the importance of gender in labour market processes (Gamarnikow 1978; Witz 1986, 1988, 1992; Walby 1989; Crompton and Sanderson 1990; Gamarnikow 1991). Witz (1992), for example, employs a neo-Weberian perspective to develop an historical analysis of the relationship between gender and professionalization in medicine, midwifery, nursing and radiography. Witz argues that gender makes a difference to both the form and the outcome of professional projects (Larson 1977). According to Witz, the patriarchal nature of the nineteenth century institutions placed severe constraints on women's ability to engage in professionalization processes. Civil society was a bastion of the male bourgeoisie. Women had to mobilize male proxy power in order to represent their collective interest at the institutional level of the state. Moreover, their exclusion from the modern university system meant they had to utilize other institutional locations for education and training. Witz argues that the disparate work and market situations of health care professionals today must be recognized as the product of past struggles by occupational groups whose access to the resources of occupational professionalism were facilitated or constrained by gender.

As Gamarnikow (1991) has shown, historically gender has been both a liability and a resource for nurses. On the one hand it has been utilized by nurses as a justification for their jurisdictional claims, on the other, it has been employed to undermine nurses' aspirations to professional status. Nineteenth century nursing reform was based on an ideological equation between nursing, femininity and women's work to which both doctors and nurses subscribed. The politics of occupational reform suggest, however, that this equation was also a political strategy employed by nursing reformers and doctors to meet different ends. The reformers' objective was to establish an occupational niche for unmarried or widowed middle-class women. They deployed explicit ideologies of femininity in an enabling manner to legitimate their jurisdictional claims. Women ought to do nursing work it was claimed, because the tasks involved were identical to those women performed in the home and because the caring qualities of the nurse were uniquely feminine. Gamarnikow (1991) argues that, by contrast, medical men defined femininity in terms of patriarchal female subordination. As the division of labour between doctors and nurses became difficult to sustain in practice, doctors used the ideologies of femininity to distinguish between dominant and subordinate forms of health care to safeguard their own position. Gamarnikow argues that although both doctors and nurses accepted a subordinate position for nurses within the health division of labour, doctors' dominance was justified on the grounds of female obedience, whereas nurses went out of their way to argue that their subordination was purely professional.

The explicit gendering of nursing as 'women's work' has made its analysis inherently problematic for feminists. On the one hand, it is possible to develop a powerful argument that women, as a result of their sex-roles, have a body of knowledge that, although largely unrecognized, is unique to their gender (Ungerson 1983). Indeed it has been suggested that the most appropriate occupational strategy for nursing is for it to be unashamedly feminine – emphasizing the unique caring and nurturing skills of women (Oakley 1984; Davies 1995). Others have cautioned against such an approach, however, arguing that it reifies gender (Gould 1988), traps women and men into gender stereotyped occupations (Savage 1987), excludes the possibility of men's involvement in caring (Ungerson 1983) and does nothing to address the devaluation of female skills (MacPherson 1991).

Gender affects not only the kinds of jobs that people do but also the rewards accruing to an occupation (Gamarnikow 1978; Davies and Rosser 1986; Rothman and Detlefs 1988; Crompton and Sanderson 1990; Gamarnikow 1991; Davies 1995). The concept of skill is far from unequivocal; it is a socially constructed concept that is intricately bound up with the sexual division of labour (Phillips and Taylor 1980). In its everyday usage it excludes much of the work done by women. Because many of the tasks in traditional female occupations are considered 'natural' for women – an extension of the feminine role – they are not classified as skilled work, they are often not classified as work at all (Needleman and Nelson 1988). An important obstacle to nursing's claims to professional status derives from the fact that most caring work is unpaid, carried out as a 'labour of love' by women in the domestic sphere. This is a major barrier to nurses arguing that they have special-ized knowledge and expertise necessitating a long theoretical as well as practical training. Examined from this perspective, the concentration of women in lower level 'professions' defined as 'semi-professions' by some theorists (Etzioni 1969) reflects their social status as women. As feminists have pointed out, the professional model is itself inherently gendered (Witz 1992; Davies 1995). Witz (1992) suggests that this is because sociological analysis has taken what are in fact successful professional projects of class-privileged male actors at a particular point in history and in particular societies and treated them as the paradigmatic case of profession. This observation has particular salience for nursing, which, as Rafferty (1996) has argued, has developed largely by analogy with the medical model of professionalism. Rafferty argues that it is ironic that the first feminist-inspired nursing elite turned to medicine as a template for the development of a professional model for nursing.

> How could a female-dominated profession succeed in advancing an agenda of self-regulation by emulating the professional tactics of the group whose dominance depends on the subordination of the group seeking independence?
>
> (Rafferty 1996: 67)

These ideas have been developed by Davies (1995) in her analysis of 'the professional predicament in nursing'. According to Davies, the discontents of nurses have to be seen in terms of a broader societal devaluation of women and the work that they do and the ways in which metaphors of masculinity have come to shape the visions of what is achieved in the health care context. Davies argues that bureaucracy and profession are important for nurses. It is common for them to berate the former and applaud the latter. Both, however, arise from an essentially masculinist vision of the world. Davies points out that the ideal decision-making of detached bureaucratic rationality and autonomous professional practice are in fact fundamentally dependent on a great deal of support work that is typically performed by women. In this respect, nurses' work has many similarities with that of secretaries (Pringle 1989) and the 'shadow-work' of women in sociology (Deegan 1995). Drawing on Pringle's (1989) work on secretaries, Davies argues:

> It is because secretaries do attend to needs that are personal, sexual and emotional, and because they carry out work that is under conceptualized, devalued and ignored, that their bosses can continue to act in a disembodied way and can continue to present their decision processes in terms of the abstract ideal that has been described.
>
> (Davies 1995: 55)

Davies maintains that the ideal-typical fleeting encounter of the consultant on the ward round is sustained in an analogous way through much preparatory and often considerable follow-up work with patients performed mainly by women. Davies concludes that there is a sense in which nursing is not a profession but an 'adjunct' to a gendered concept of profession. Nursing is the activity that enables medicine to present itself as masculine/rational and to gain the power and the privilege of doing so. Davies suggests that the problems of nursing need to be considered as deriving from the efforts of the leaders of the occupation to put a conceptual frame around those aspects of the work of health and healing that are 'left over' after medicine has imposed an essentially masculinist vision.

Similar themes are developed by Wicks (1998), who argues that nursing is constituted through a 'duality of focus', comprised, on the one hand, of the goals of nursing practice and, on the other, the political reality of nursing positioned as it is in a 'network of scientific power'. 'This was expressed by one nurse in the conflicting imperatives expressed concerning "getting through the 2.00 p.m. observations", and wanting to sit and talk with a lonely and anxious patient who clearly needed the comfort of contact' (Wicks 1998: 172).

Both Davies and Wicks provide fascinating insights into the gendering of nursing work. Nevertheless, at times, they are guilty of overstating their respective positions. Wicks (1998), for example, appears to present the political position of nursing purely in terms of the gendered division of labour between doctors and nurses. But as I have argued in Chapter 1, economic interests have also been a significant force in fashioning the shape of nursing work.

The part played by capital and patriarchy in producing sexual inequality has been a central concern in feminist theorizing. Bradley (1989) and Walby (1986) provide useful overviews. Bradley (1989) discusses this literature in terms of a continuum. At one extreme, traditional Marxists have argued that gender divisions could be explained within a general theory of class. These approaches have tended to see the position of women purely in terms of the needs of capital: they have little to say about gender relations *per se* (Walby 1986) and fail to see that men as a social group might benefit from the position of women (Walby 1986; Bradley 1989). At the other end of the spectrum, radical feminists have concentrated on the analysis of patriarchy. The concept of patriarchy has proven difficult to define, however, and has tended to be used in a vague way to refer to male dominance in every form.

Most feminists agree that neither capital nor patriarchy alone adequately account for gender inequalities and more recently debates have centred on the nature of the relations between the two. Some have argued that capitalism and patriarchal relations are so entwined that they form a mutually interdependent system (Eisenstein 1979; cited by Walby 1986). Others have argued for the development of a dual systems approach – in which capitalism and patriarchy are separate but interacting systems. Advocates of the dual systems approach argue that class cannot be reduced to gender or gender to class, and that the two should be theorized separately but that at any historical moment they are found interacting. The precise character of their articulation is, however, subject to debate. Some have assumed relatively harmonious relations between capital and patriarchy (Hartmann 1979; Hartmann 1981; cited by Walby 1986), whereas others have highlighted the ways in which the two systems can be in tension and conflict (Walby 1986). Witz (1992) has employed a dual systems approach in her analysis of female professional projects within the health division of labour. I have already delineated Witz's observations on the significance of gender in shaping the process and the outcome of women's professional projects in the health care context. She also underlines the importance of powerful economic interests in resisting nursing reform and moulding the structure it was to eventually assume.

Taken together, the writings of Hughes, Durkheim, Abbott and feminist scholars provide a framework that can be utilized in the study of nursing. Their main contribution is to our understanding of nursing's occupational status within the division of labour in society as a whole; however, they do not provide an adequate theoretical basis for analysing the ways in which nurses manage their occupational boundaries in the work setting, although they clearly consider work place processes to be important. For this we must look to theories of social interaction.

The division of labour as social interaction

As Freidson (1976) has argued, at the most fundamental level, the ultimate reality of the division of labour lies in the social interaction of its participants.

> [I]n the everyday world of work from which we abstract conceptions of the division of labor, it seems accurate to see the division of labor as a process of social interaction in the course of which the participants are continuously engaged in attempting to define, establish, maintain and renew the tasks they perform and the relationship with others which their tasks presuppose.
>
> (Freidson 1976: 311)

Freidson is keen to emphasize that such interaction is not entirely free and individual, rather it is constrained in complex ways by, for example, variations in power on the part of the participants as well as by the characteristics of the material world. The nature of the relationship between freedom and constraints in social life has preoccupied social theorists for a long time and the relative importance of social structure and human agency has been fiercely debated within sociology (see, for example, Dawe 1970). One important attempt to transcend this distinction is the negotiated order perspective (cf. Berger and Luckman 1967; Giddens 1984).

Negotiated order perspective

The term 'negotiated order' was introduced into the literature by Strauss *et al.* (1963, 1964) as a way of conceptualizing the ordered flux they found in their study of two North American psychiatric hospitals between 1958 and 1962 (Maines 1982). Strauss *et al.* (1963) argued that hitherto, students of formal organizations had tended to over-emphasize stable structures and formal rules at the expense of internal change. It was suggested that a more fruitful approach would be to conceptualize the social order as in process, reconstituted continually through myriad processes of social interaction. The negotiated order theorists attempted to show how social interaction (negotiation) contributes to the constitution of social orders (structures) and how social orders give form to interaction processes (Maines 1982).

The nature of this relationship has been a key issue in the development of the paradigm. For example, a frequent charge is that the approach assumes everything is indefinitely negotiable and is thus unable to deal with limiting factors in social settings (Benson 1977a,b, 1978; Day and Day 1977, 1978; Dingwall and Strong 1985). It is certainly possible to find passages in Strauss' early writings to support such a criticism.

> The realm of rules could then be usefully pictured as a tiny island of structured stability around which swirled and beat a vast ocean of negotiation. But we could push the metaphor further and assert what is already implicit in our discussion: that there is *only* vast ocean.
>
> (Strauss *et al*. 1964: 313)

Closer inspection of the early texts suggest, however, that Strauss *et al*. did not discard the notion of constraint as unequivocally as their critics claim. For example, reference is made to organizational hierarchies shaping patterns of negotiation (Strauss *et al*. 1964: 304) and the constraining effects of formal policies and rules (Strauss *et al*. 1964: 313). In later work, moreover, Strauss (1978) introduces the concepts of 'negotiation context' and 'structural context' to sensitize researchers to the relationship between negotiation processes and extra-situational constraint arguing that:

> [N]ot everything is either equally negotiable or – at any given time or period of time – negotiable at all. One of the researcher's main tasks, as it is that of the negotiating parties themselves, is to discover just what is negotiable at any given time.
>
> (Strauss 1978: 252)

A number of studies have subsequently attempted to examine the dialectic between structural constraints and negotiation processes (see, for example, *Urban Life* Special Edition – October 1982). Busch's (1982) analysis shows the historical processes through which structural conditions are produced by negotiations and, once produced, shape subsequent negotiations. Hall and Spencer-Hall's (1982) comparison of two North American public school systems suggests ways in which different organizational arrangements suppress or encourage negotiations. Sugrue (1982) described the effects of emotions, and Kleinman (1982) examines the import of actors' theories of negotiations, on negotiation processes. Levy (1982) employs a dramaturgical perspective and introduces the concept of 'staging' in order to describe the mechanisms through which the various parties to negotiations attempt to alter the negotiation context to secure their desired outcomes, for example, by attempting to gain control over organizational rules and ground rules.

More recently, this theme has been taken up by Svensson (1996) in his study of the interplay between doctors and nurses. Drawing on interview data with nursing staff on medical and surgical wards in five Swedish hospitals, Svensson claims that the conditions for inter-occupational negotiation have altered fundamentally over the past decade, augmenting the influence of nurses vis-à-vis doctors. He argues that viewed in historical terms, the relationship between doctors and nurses has 'changed dramatically'. Svensson attributes this shift in the doctor–nurse relationship to three key changes in the negotiation context that have given nurses 'space' for directly influencing patient care decisions and interpreting organizational rules. First, he argues that the increased prevalence of chronic illness has resulted in a shift of emphasis from preventing death to handling life, introducing a social dimension into health care. According to Svensson, nurses are powerfully placed to contribute to patient management given the centrality of 'the social' to holistic care. Second, Svensson maintains that the shift from a system of task allocation to team nursing has fundamentally altered the nurse–doctor relationship. Team-nursing facilitates a closer nurse–patient relationship because the nurse is responsible for fewer patients. Moreover, the nurse's knowledge of the patient is no longer exchanged in a two-step process via the ward sister, but presented directly to the doctor. Third, Svensson argues that the introduction on many wards of the sitting round, where the doctor and nurse discuss their patients before the 'walking' round, offers an arena in which nurses feel more able to converse with the doctor and influence patient management decisions.

Svensson's work is an important contribution to sociological understanding of contemporary doctor–nurse interaction and also to the relationship between negotiation processes and social orders. Unfortunately, as Svensson himself concedes, the analysis is hamstrung by its reliance on interview data that cannot necessarily be read as literal descriptions of an external reality (Scott and Lyman 1968; Silverman 1993: 90–114). Moreover, although Svensson is concerned with the patterns of interaction between doctors *and* nurses, the interviews were undertaken with nurses only, and thus we are given only a partial view. This raises the question as to whether nurses' position has shifted as radically as Svensson claims. Acknowledging some of the shortcomings of his data, Svensson suggests that one way in which sociological analysis of the ward as a negotiated order could be further developed is through the utilization of systematic observational methods.

'Doing' nursing jurisdiction

In developing the negotiated order perspective in the context of this study I have adopted a broad conceptualization of extra-situational constraint, including actors' orientations to social structures, the immediate interactional context, practical and material constraints, macrosociological considerations such as gender, and wider organizational factors, as well as historical and political considerations. I have also endeavoured to augment the approach by following the lead of ethnomethodology and paying close attention to members' talk. For, as Heritage observes, at its most fundamental level, social reality is talked into being (Heritage 1984). As Mellinger (1994) has pointed out, however, although the negotiated order perspective has significantly enhanced our understanding of occupational settings, little attention has been given to the properties of real world negotiations. As well as offering access to actors' formulations of organizational structures and constraints, an approach that attends to 'talk' offers clear methodological advantages in that one's empirical observations can be reproduced, others can do further analysis and potentially challenge the analysts' interpretation of events.

Attending to the formative powers of talk raises the question of how to operationalize the concept of negotiation in an empirical study. What do negotiations look like and where can they be found? A commonsense understanding of the notion of negotiation suggests a direct interactional exchange of some kind that ought to yield the types of textual data favoured by an ethnomethodological approach. In the literature, however, the concept of negotiation is poorly defined. It is used to refer to 'bargaining, compromising, brokering, mediating or collusion' (Maines 1977), 'making a deal (an explicit compromise), trading off, reaching an informal agreement (say with respect to each other's turf), or reaching more formal agreements signified by contracts and other signed arrangements' (Strauss 1978). Negotiations can be one-shot or serial and carried out over a variable time scale (Strauss 1978). Most significantly, Strauss also indicates that negotiations may be unspoken or tacit (Strauss *et al.* 1964). This clearly raises important methodological problems for researchers committed to a focus on talk and text and, as we will see, this is an issue that has particular relevance for the negotiation of nursing jurisdiction. Given these considerations therefore, I prefer to consider the social order as continuously accomplished or 'done' rather than negotiated. This entails retaining the foundational assumptions of the negotiated order perspective – that social reality is the product of the meaningful actions of actors – but employs a broader approach to reality construction, in which negotiations (defined as an interactional exchange of text or talk) are one of a number of possible processes through which the social world is produced (Allen 1997a). Such an approach indicates the need for a research methodology that combines an ethnomethodological interest in talk with more orthodox ethnographic concerns.

Summary and conclusion

In this chapter I have considered in some detail a number of sociological theories and identified key threads that may be usefully woven together in the study of nursing work. To recapitulate, my aim was to develop a non-essentialist conceptualization of nursing that enabled us to comprehend the occupation's location within an overall societal division of labour, but that also permitted an appreciation of the intricate detail of the social production of nursing work on hospital wards and in other locales. In the framework I have proposed the societal division of labour is conceived of as a social system. Work is defined as the activities that need to be done in a given society and is not limited to paid work in the public sphere. The world of work is dynamic. System disturbance may arise from a number of sources: social, technological, economic and organizational change. Because the system of work is constantly in flux, occupations change. Jurisdictions expand and contract and the boundaries between paid and unpaid work domains may shift. New occupations emerge, others fuse and some may decline or disappear totally. The value and status of activities undertaken by an occupation may be modified. It is against this ever-changing world that occupations vie to secure their standing. One of the ways in which they can do this is by claiming professional status. As we have seen, certain segments of the nursing body are currently engaged in just this kind of process.

Although it may exhibit certain stable features, the division of labour is, at its base, the product of diverse processes of social interaction in public, legal and workplace arenas. Put in another way, occupational boundaries are not self evident, they have to be actively constructed and reconstructed by the participants concerned. The interactional accomplishment of occupational boundaries does not take place in a vacuum, however, it is shaped by wider structural constraints: material and practical conditions, historical and political considerations, organizational factors, the immediate interactional context and macrosociological conditions, of which, in the case of nursing, gender and economics are the most important.

3

THE STUDY

The research took place over a 10-month period and focused on two wards at Woodlands District General Hospital: Treetops, a thirty-three-bedded surgical ward, and Fernlea, a thirty-four-bedded medical unit. Ethnographic methods were employed. The data comprise fieldnotes and audio-tape recordings derived from participant observation in the study site (including 12 weeks, intensive observation on each ward); tape-recorded semi-structured interviews with a sample of nurses, doctors, auxiliaries, health care assistants and clinical managers, and the analysis of documentary evidence.

This chapter introduces the research site and discusses how the data were generated. The collection and analysis of data on the research process forms part of a distinctive methodology most explicitly developed in the writings of Hammersley and Atkinson (1983) and which finds expression in the notion of reflexivity. It is a methodological stance that cuts through the well-rehearsed polemics between positivism and naturalism. It is, they argue, an unavoidable existential fact, that we are part of the world we study. Rather than trying to avoid the effects of the researcher on the study setting, therefore, we should endeavour to better understand them. Reflexivity underlines the role of the researcher as an active generator of data, engaged as s/he is in the processes of interpretation and pattern making common to everyday social life. It is the researcher who must decide what to observe, who to talk to, what questions to ask and how to interpret events. Understanding the processes through which the research data were generated and the assumptions that guided the choices that were made is a central mechanism through which the validity and reliability of the research findings can be assessed.

Guiding assumptions
As outlined in Chapter 2, the study was guided by a non-essentialist conceptualization of the nursing role. I started with the assumption

that the world of work was a dynamic social system in which occupations and their boundaries were constantly changing and evolving in response to a range of external factors. From this perspective then, nursing jurisdiction is historically contingent, that is, there is no necessary relationship between the occupational category 'nurse' and the bundle of tasks (Hughes 1984) that adhere to the title. Rather, a 'nurse' is what people called 'nurses' do in a given historical context (Dingwall 1983a,b). I have suggested that over the course of its occupational development, nursing jurisdiction has been shaped by a complex configuration of social, technological, organizational and economic factors, the effects of which have been mediated in a variety of arenas by the discourses of professionalism and managerialism. This research was undertaken against the backdrop of developments in nursing and medical education and health policy that had precipitated a revival of these historical tensions, creating jurisdictional ambiguity for practitioners. I have argued that although they are clearly important, ultimately they are only ideas about nursing work. At a more fundamental level, the actual division of labour is produced through numerous processes of social interaction, in other words, nurses have to 'do' jurisdiction. My aim in undertaking this study was to move on from the policy debates to explore the ways in which nurses were producing the boundaries of their practice in the course of their routine work.

The hospital

Woodlands hospital is a district general hospital in the middle of England. At the time of the study it had almost 900 beds, an annual budget of £60 million, 2,800 employees and provided general, acute, obstetric and elderly services to a local population of 254,000. Situated in a tightly integrated community in what was once a major industrial area, Woodlands was the largest employer in a locality blighted by high levels of unemployment. For over two centuries heavy industry had been the principal employment in the town. Between 1978 and 1987 more than 8,000 jobs had been lost and much of the industry had gone forever. A pristine 'out-of-town' shopping complex now stands where once (mainly) men laboured, and local shoppers had witnessed the replacement of 'high street' names with discount shops in the town centre. In 1995, a report on poverty undertaken by the Borough Council's Anti-Poverty Unit revealed unemployment in the area to be 16 per cent (about 6 per cent higher than the national average), with local employers offering some of the lowest rates of pay in the country. Over

4,000 jobs had been lost between 1990 and 1995, leaving 20,000 people without work (8 per cent of the total local population). More than 55,000 (22 per cent) of local people were receiving state income support. Many of the women working in the hospital were the principal breadwinners in their households – a significant role reversal in a traditional working class community.

Woodlands was a *local* hospital. Its stated aim was to provide the best in hospital care for the immediate community and it drew on the indigenous population for most of its non-medical staff. Few of the nurses who trained at the hospital came from outside the immediate area. Nurses who did not train in the hospital never quite fitted in, it was felt.

> *I'm an outsider even though I've been here a long time. I didn't train here so I'm an outsider.*
>
> (Nurse Manager)

Like the local community it served, Woodlands had a cohesive organizational culture. Hospital employees included many members of the same family and hospital-wide activities – staff lottery, art competition, summer fete and annual outing – aimed to further facilitate social integration. This close knit culture was variously experienced as friendly or oppressive depending on one's viewpoint.

> *I like it because it's not big. You know most of the people in the canteen or if you don't they'll always say hello to you. Like I smoke [...] You can always find somebody to sit and have a natter with. It seems quite sociable.*
>
> (Staff Nurse)

She [EN] explained that [...] the pregnancy was not planned. She said that she had needed time to 'get her head round it' herself so she did not tell anyone. This hospital is such a gossipy place, she said, I decided I couldn't deal with people questioning me so I didn't tell anyone.

My first contact with Woodlands was four years before the study began. On this occasion the encounter was brief and, preoccupied as I was with the well-being of my son, I retained few lasting impressions. The hospital seemed much the same as others in which I had worked in the preceding seven years. Returning four years later, however, things appeared very different. In the intervening period the hospital had witnessed large-scale organizational changes heralded by the 1990 NHS and Community Care Act. The thread most evident on revisiting the hospital was the consumerist emphasis. Woodlands did not *look* like the hospitals I was familiar with. Soothing pink wallcoverings and co-ordinating floral borders had replaced the, once ubiquitous, eggshell emulsion and the floors were carpeted, albeit only in places. Staff smiled benevolently from photoboards, interspersed at intervals by quality assurance notices and suggestion boxes. This was the outpatients department, however, the shop window of the hospital and, as I was to discover, generally regarded as something of a showpiece. Moving further into the building the sights became more familiar. I discovered a restaurant with its daily menu chalked on a blackboard outside the entrance. Inside, fluorescent strip lighting revealed orange plastic chairs arranged around chipped Formica tables. This was a scene altogether more reminiscent of the hospitals in which I had worked. The contrast with the outpatients department was striking and just one example of the ways in which symbols of the old and new order were regularly juxtaposed throughout the hospital.

Considerable effort had been expended promoting a slick corporate image. Woodlands employed its own marketing manager, and as the fieldwork progressed, I became aware of the variety of ways in which the organization was promoted, both locally on hospital vehicles, badges and public information literature and, more widely, in the glossy folders sent to prospective employees. Clinical staff were frequently derisory about the effort put into organizational 'impression management' (Goffman 1959).

> As I sat at the table at the far end of the ward this morning I overheard the EN talking to the patients about the hospital and the NHS. She was complaining about the ways in which the hospital chose to spend its money 'on posh carpets and things like that rather than on things for the patients'.

Along with two other local hospitals, Woodlands had formed an NHS Trust in 1993, delivering services previously provided by the General Hospitals Unit that it replaced. A system of eleven clinical directorates had been established and key management functions devolved. This merged the management arrangements for all three hospitals. At the time the study was undertaken, clinical directors controlled over 65 per cent of Trust expenditure and there were plans for further devolution. Each directorate had a clinical management team that was headed by the clinical director who was a consultant, and also included a general manager, nurse manager and accountant. The clinical directors were members of the Trust management board.

The wards

Treetops was a mixed-sex urology ward. Its population comprised patients (mainly men) undergoing surgery or investigation of the prostate gland or bladder, and, less commonly, those who had had surgical removal of a kidney or the bladder. Although managed by the surgical directorate, people suffering from conditions where no immediate surgery was indicated were also accommodated. The ward also cared for patients in the terminal stages of bladder or prostate cancer. Fernlea was a mixed-sex ward too, but its patient population was clinically more varied. Ten beds were allocated to rheumatology cases and the remaining twenty-four to acute medical conditions, such as cardiac, respiratory, vascular and gastric disorders.

At Woodlands, there were four wards on each floor, which ran end-to-end along one side of the main hospital building. Access from the main hospital thoroughfare was via two connecting corridors where a ward stretched out at right angles on either side. The only boundary marker between the wards was a shared entrance lobby where two steel linen trolleys stared at each other blankly from under half open tarpaulin covers. Physically identical, each ward was arranged around a central corridor. Along one side were five, six-bedded patient areas separated from the main ward corridor by a partially glazed panel. Opposite were the toilet and bathrooms, the patients' sitting room, and three other single-bedded rooms (on Treetops one of these had been converted into an office for use by the nurse practitioner). The central corridor was flanked by pieces of equipment partially shrouded by old counterpanes, and the wall opposite the patient areas was lined with public information notices. The focal point of the ward was the nurses' station which was opposite the first patient bay. The sluice lay behind to the right and, to the left was a small recess, which housed the ward computer, drugs trolley and refrigerator. This was a 'back-stage' area (Goffman 1959) – the only space on the ward where patients were not permitted access – and it was here that nurses and support staff would retreat for an informal break if workload pressures permitted.

The wards had rather different rates of patient turnover. Patient throughput on Treetops was relatively rapid. According to the ward activity analysis figures, average length of stay was 5.1 days during the fieldwork period compared with 8 days on Fernlea. Pressure on medical beds was intense, whereas empty beds were fairly common on the surgical ward. Fernlea's average daily bed occupancy during the fieldwork period was thirty-one out of a total bed availability of thirty-four, compared to twenty-two out of a daily bed availability of thirty-three on Treetops.[1]

The work environment on Treetops was characterized by dramatic changes in the pace of activity. During the week the nurses' daily work rhythms were marked by periods of frenetic activity punctuated by lulls. An atmosphere of busyness was associated with the daily theatre operating schedules – either the processing and preparation of patients for theatre or their close monitoring in the immediate post-operative period. Patients went to surgery every day of the week and beds were regularly moved in order to allocate those patients who had most recently undergone surgery to high dependency spaces. Weekends were comparatively quiet, however, and nurses used this time to prepare paperwork for the next week's routine admissions.

The pace of work was steadier on Fernlea. There were certainly peaks and troughs of activity but these tended to be related to unforeseen changes in the condition of patients, rather than the demands of external organizational timetables as was the case on Treetops.

> Saturday it was like a nursing home. They were all well. There was only Mrs Daley who was unwell. Then Sunday it was more like ITU [intensive care unit]! They've all got PEs [pulmonary embolism] it seems.
>
> (Senior Sister)

Furthermore, the contrast between the work rhythms on weekdays and weekends was not as marked as it was on the surgical ward.

Both wards were staffed by a combination of nurses, support workers and students in training. On Treetops the team comprised: the ward manager, a junior sister, two senior staff nurses, ten junior staff nurses, one enrolled nurse, three health care assistants and three nursing auxiliaries. All the auxiliaries worked part-time and only one of the health care assistants worked full-time. One of the junior staff nurses worked part-time and was employed on a 6-month contract. Final year student nurses had placements on the ward and were included in the staffing levels. During the period of my fieldwork there were two groups of students on the ward (five in the first and three in the second). Medical staff comprised one permanent and one locum consultant urologist, and two senior house officers (SHOs). The senior house officers shared the ward work with a nurse practitioner whose post had been funded through the junior doctors' hours initiative (NHSME 1991).

The Fernlea nursing team included: a ward manager, a junior sister, two senior staff nurses, eight junior staff nurses, one health care assistant and three auxiliaries. One auxiliary and one junior staff nurse worked part-time. The ward had final year students who were also included in the staffing numbers. There were two groups of students on the ward during the period of the fieldwork (three in each). The general medical team comprised: the consultant, registrar, SHO and junior house officer (HO). The rheumatology team comprised a consultant, staff grade doctor and SHO.

Table 1

	Number of staff	
	Treetops	*Fernlea*
Ward Manager	1	1
Junior Sister	1	1
Senior Staff Nurse	2	2
Junior Staff Nurse	10	8
Enrolled Nurse	1	–
HCA	3	1
Auxiliary Nurse	3	3
Student Nurse	5/3	3/3
Consultant	2	2
Registrar	–	1
SHO	2	2
HO	–	1
Nurse Practitioner	1	-
Staff Grade Doctor	–	1

Negotiating access

Initial access

Research access was negotiated through the Director of Nursing who, after an initial telephone conversation, agreed to meet in order to discuss the possibility of taking the research forward. The date of the meeting was confirmed in a letter and an outline of the research was enclosed (see Allen 1996). When the meeting took place the Director of Nursing immediately offered her support for the study and explained that the Director of Medicine had also approved the research plan. It was suggested that I attended the next senior nurses' meeting in order to begin the process of communicating the details of the research to the study participants. I was also introduced to Debbie – the nurse manager responsible for clinical audit – who was nominated to act as an organizational 'link-person'. Although herself a relatively new addition to the hospital staff, she proved a valuable contact, providing important background information about the hospital, suggesting people to talk to and making several introductions. Through Debbie I also established two further key informants. Greta had responsibility for the implementation of Project 2000 and was involved in general professional development issues. She was an important link with the health care assistants as she was responsible for their training and it was through her that I was able to attend a variety of in-service training days. Pauline was another key informant. Her remit was tissue viability. She had trained at Woodlands, had good clinical links and was identified as someone who 'knew all the gossip'.

Negotiating access to the wards

Treetops

At the suggestion of the Director of Nursing I began the study on Treetops. The ward was identified as suitable because they had recently employed a nurse practitioner in a role that was perceived to cross traditional occupational boundaries. I also had a preference for urology as I had recent clinical experience of this speciality, which I felt would be a useful interactional resource. Access was negotiated through the two ward sisters who agreed to meet with me to discuss the project.

My first contact with the ward was a telephone call to the senior sister in order to set a date for a meeting. Although she agreed to meet me her tone indicated a degree of reluctance.

> If they've said you can do it here, then really we have to accommodate you dear. As long as you keep out of our way when we're busy.
>
> (Sister)

Our conversation left me feeling bemused, and raised important ethical dilemmas around the notion of consent. Formal access had already been granted by powerful individuals within the organization, but the ward sister made it clear she felt unable to refuse access without incurring official censure. Without her support for the work, however, it was hard to see how access could be achieved in any meaningful sense.

I eventually met with the ward sisters to discuss taking the study forward. A key objective of the meeting was to gain their trust by establishing myself as an honest and decent person who possessed sufficient 'native wit' to not make unreasonable demands on the ward staff. The meeting was a strange event. The sisters were both very friendly and welcoming but I found it frustratingly difficult to give anything like the comprehensive account of the research I had planned to do. They were clearly eager to give me the information they felt I needed and I had to perform a delicate interactional balancing act to ensure that I had fully explained the research without appearing uninterested in what they had to say. On reflection, however, it is clear that we had come to the meeting with quite different agendas. My aim was to give a full account of the study to ensure that the research was taken forward on sound ethical grounds, but as far as the sisters were concerned, research was a rather esoteric business carried out by 'very clever' people that neither interested or concerned them. Furthermore, they were already resigned to the fact that the research would be taken forward on the unit; and, having reached this point, saw the meeting as an opportunity to discuss the practical implications of the research for the staff and to make it clear that the ward was a busy one and that I was not to get in the way.

I gave the senior ward sister copies of the research outline to distribute to all nursing staff, stressing that auxiliaries and HCAs should also receive one. Yet while she agreed to my request, it was evident that she regarded it as rather unorthodox. I left the meeting unconvinced she would do as she promised but was unable to pursue the issue further without straining friendly relations. In actuality, the support staff were never given any information about the research, not even verbally. I explained that I had left outlines for them, but they must have been over-looked. The support staff expressed no surprise that they had not been informed about the project and the incident did not appear to damage my relationships with them in anyway. The event proved to be an early sign of the strength of the nursing hierarchy on the ward and was in marked contrast to my experiences in negotiating access to the medical ward.

Fernlea

Access to Fernlea was negotiated through Pauline, who had herself been a sister on the ward. She arranged a meeting with the ward sister and facilitated the process by explaining my study and vouching for my personal acceptability. I met with the junior sister, who explained that the senior sister was unable to join us but was happy for the study to go ahead. Although I did not appreciate it at the time, this was an early indication of the division of labour between the two sisters on the ward, which was an on-going source of strain.

This meeting was easier than the one on the surgical ward but there were important differences between the two events. The second meeting was dyadic rather than a triadic exchange and by this time I had been a participant observer at the hospital for three months and had first-hand knowledge of what the fieldwork would mean for the staff. Like the sisters on Treetops, the medical sister was chiefly concerned with the practical implications of the work rather than the details of the study itself, but at this stage in the research I had come to expect this as normal. The sister was happy for the study to go ahead but first wanted to meet with the rest of the ward staff – nursing, medical and support workers – in order to explain the research details. This consultation process ended up being rather protracted: I made contact on a number of occasions and was informed by the senior sister that negotiations were no further forward. Eventually I made a spontaneous decision to visit the ward when I was in the hospital for another purpose. I met with the junior sister who informed me that although she had not had an opportunity to discuss the project with everyone she did not envisage that there would be any problems. A start date was arranged and when I eventually began the fieldwork a copy of the research outline was pinned on the notice board and all staff knew about the research, even if they were not acquainted with its finer details.

Night staff

On both wards separate negotiations were undertaken with night staff. This entailed sending the nursing managers copies of the research outline and making contact by telephone in order to introduce myself. I purposively scheduled my routine observations on the wards to overlap with the night shift in order that I could make myself known and explain the purposes of the study.

Data generation

Observations and participation

As Hammersley and Atkinson (1983) point out, having selected the case(s) for ethnographic study, decisions must also be made about what one is going to observe. I was eager to understand the perspective of all those involved in the social construction of nursing jurisdiction, and this included clinicians involved in the daily negotiation of work boundaries – doctors, support workers and nurses themselves – as well as clinical managers concerned with formal organizational policy. Moreover, I wanted to develop an understanding of how occupational boundaries were negotiated in the different arenas of the organization.

A thorough grounding in the ethnographic literature on hospitals (Hughes and Allen 1993a) and my nursing experience meant that I began the research with some idea about which aspects of ward life were likely to yield data relevant to the research question. These were nursing handover, ward rounds, ward meetings, the introduction of new staff to the ward, administration of medications, work allocation, admission and discharge processes, interaction at the nurses' station, interaction in 'back-stage' regions, and interaction between staff when the patient was and was not present. I anticipated that this initial strategy would be modified as the research progressed in accordance with my developing theoretical concerns.

Time is an important feature of hospital social organization (Zerubavel 1979) and fieldwork was organized in order to sample the major temporal divisions. I planned to spend four hours in the field, on three days each week. Observations were scheduled to cover 06:00–10:00, 10:00–14:00, 14:00–18:00, and 18:00–22:00 for each day of the week. On a number of occasions I spent whole shifts on the ward and I also observed four separate night shifts. My preparedness to work unsociable hours was met with approval by the study participants and did much to demonstrate my sincerity and commitment to understanding their work.

Under the guidance of the Director of Nursing, I wore a white coat in the ward areas. Like other white-coat-wearers at the hospital I left this unbuttoned and so it was necessary to give some thought to what I wore underneath. I adopted a style of dress with which I felt personally comfortable and that was in keeping with the broad dress codes of non-uniformed personnel within the hospital: smart casual. I was also provided with a badge that carried the hospital logo and on which I elected to have inscribed – 'Davina Allen Research Student'. I purposely avoided using 'nurse' in the title to avoid misleading patients and organizational members as to my role.

I was clear that I did not want to work as a qualified nurse. As well as lacking confidence in my clinical skills, I felt this would restrict my access to certain groups, limit the activities I would be able to observe, and make it difficult to stick to my plan of keeping detailed fieldnotes of participants' talk (see Chapter 2). In the early stages of the study, however, I spontaneously volunteered to do things without giving any consideration to my ability to carry them through. In part, this reflected my discomfiture with the research role, which was new to me, but it was also an indicator of my own dis-ease with being on the ward and not contributing to 'getting through the work' (Clarke 1978). As the fieldwork progressed, however, I was able to negotiate a social niche I felt more comfortable with and that could be adapted to my purposes. This had three main elements: researcher as 'helper', researcher as 'observer', and researcher as 'shadow'.

Sometimes I involved myself closely with the ward work. I answered the telephone, relayed messages to staff and to relatives, gave out meals and drinks, assisted with toiletting, made patients comfortable, disposed of bedpans and urinals, lent books, provided bibliographic references for students, chaperoned male doctors examining female patients, and acted as a 'go-fer' for both nursing and medical staff. Nevertheless, it was an on-going dilemma as to how involved to become in the ward work without being perceived by the nursing staff to be interfering and I had to make largely intuitive judgements according to the context.

On other occasions I adopted more of an observer role, positioning myself in a strategic spot in order to watch the ebb-and-flow of ward activities. The nurses' station proved a useful vantage point, as it was here that much of the work activity was co-ordinated. By locating myself in this area I was able to observe the division of labour at work and transcribe members' talk directly into my notebook.

The third strategy I employed was to shadow participants in their everyday work. I spent periods of up to 14 hours with the on-call doctors in a style of observation that might best be described as 'a-day-in-the-life-of'. As I shall outline in Chapter 7, the work of doctors and nurses has a different spatial and geographic organization, and shadowing medical staff in this way provided access to those aspects of medical work that are largely invisible to ward-based staff. In the early stages of the research I attempted to shadow a single nurse in the same way as I had the doctors, but I found this almost impossible to sustain because I felt such an encumbrance. So, rather than focusing on individual nurses, I elected to observe nursing activities such as, patient processing, escorting patients to and from theatre, technical procedures, nursing handover, work allocation, liaising with medical staff, tidying the ward, drugs administration, care-planning and record-keeping. Although I did not shadow HCAs and auxiliaries, much of the work in which I was involved on the wards were tasks that were routinely allocated to them.

Although the field role I negotiated enabled me to experience the division of labour at work and gain an understanding of the perspectives of the major occupational groups in this study, it did restrict my access to those aspects of caring work that take place 'behind the screens' (Lawler 1991). I felt that without a caring purpose it was illegitimate for me to intrude into patients' privacy.

In addition to the ward-based observations, data were also generated through attendance at nursing and management meetings and in-service study days that were tape-recorded where permitted.

Interviews

The observational data were supplemented by fifty-seven tape-recorded interviews carried out with ward nurses ($n = 29$), doctors ($n = 8$), auxiliaries ($n = 5$), health care assistants ($n = 3$) and clinical managers ($n = 11$).[2] The length of each interview ranged from 30 minutes to 3.5 hours, although typically they lasted between 30–90 minutes. In most cases, they took place in private spaces away from the main working areas. The interviews may be best described as semi-focused. I had a set of topics I wanted to discuss but no standardized questions as such, although certain questions became more-or-less routine for particular groups as the research progressed.

I had hoped that the interviews would have a conversational flavour and indeed many of them did. Some were interactionally difficult, however, and more closely resembled a job interview, with respondents clearly anxious to be giving the 'right' answer. This was particularly the case with support staff but it was also true of some of the nurses as well. However hard I tried to define the interview situation as an informal occasion – 'as just an opportunity to have a chat away from the ward' – and despite explaining to staff that there were no 'right' answers, this was not always the way in which it was perceived. I found these interviews personally very unsettling and was grateful that they characterized only a minority of those I carried out.

It is commonplace for methodology textbooks to emphasize the importance of establishing rapport with the interviewee before the interview takes place, but little has been written about the interview's impact on subsequent field relations when – as is the case in ethnography – interviews are not isolated interactional events. Because I wanted to use my observations to shape the questions I asked staff, I had postponed the interviews until a month into the fieldwork. Moreover, I felt that by this time I would have established a rapport with the research participants. The nurses clearly discussed the interviews amongst themselves, however, and, as their informal style and non-threatening nature became common knowledge, my field relationships significantly improved. As a consequence, I began my interviews with the nursing and support workers at a much earlier stage on the second ward.

Nurses and support staff often used the interview as an opportunity to discuss interpersonal difficulties and on several occasions I turned my tape-recorder off when staff became overwhelmed by the strength of their feelings. I did not consider myself to be researching a sensitive subject and was quite unprepared for this. Not only were these interviews emotionally exhausting, but cast as counsellor or agony aunt, I was unable to address the issues I wanted to discuss for the purposes of the research, indeed to have to attempted to do so would have been utterly parasitic. As the fieldwork progressed and I became more enmeshed in this complex web of relationships I experienced tremendous personal discomfort about different members' disclosures.

I also carried out informal interviews. These took the form of spontaneous extended conversations that were not tape-recorded, but that were more detailed and reflective than the briefer discussions I had with staff as they worked. Much of the data generated on the medical perspective came from interactions of this kind.

Documents

I have also drawn on a wide range of organizational literature: formal public documents (patient information leaflets and strategic documents such as the hospital's application for Trust status); formal internal literature (policy documents, job descriptions, minutes from meetings, memoranda, the hospital newspaper, duty rotas, team brief, ward philosophies, quality monitoring documents, medical and nursing records); and informal organizational texts (staff notice-boards, communication notes between staff, ward round books, and ward diaries).

Data management and analysis

Field observations were recorded in a spiral-bound shorthand notebook. Notes were taken either contemporaneously or as soon as possible after the event. These were subsequently transcribed and elaborated upon, usually the same or the next day. Key findings of each field contact and their relationship to my developing theoretical ideas were recorded on a 'contact summary' *pro forma* (Miles and Huberman 1994). Analytical ideas were documented in a separate file of memos. In another 'strategy' file I made notes on the practical implications of the work – what to see, who to talk to, which meetings to negotiate access to etc. As Dey (1993) has argued, qualitative data analysis requires a dialectic between ideas and data analysis. This dialectic informs data analysis from the outset, rendering arguments about whether data analysis is based on deduction or induction redundant. Although I began this study with a clear idea about the research focus, I was quite prepared to modify this according to the themes emerging from the field.

Over the course of the study, the style of my fieldnotes changed. Initially I made abstract and generalized notes on lots of things but as the research became more focused my notes became more detailed. I recorded naturally occurring talk on those samples of social interaction that were central to the developing research themes. I employed a behaviourist approach, that is, I utilized low-inference descriptors and attempted to record conversations verbatim. I also adopted a policy of keeping observations separate from my personal feelings, although I did not always succeed. In addition I made tape-recordings of interviews, meetings, study days, nursing handover and ward rounds. Tape-recordings of nursing handover and ward rounds were completely transcribed. Initially, interviews were completely transcribed, but as the developing themes of the research began to emerge this was limited to relevant sections only. A note was made of the content of non-transcribed material in order to provide a sense of the context for the transcribed data and enable me to easily identify material that I may have wanted to return to. I listened and re-listened to tape-recordings of meetings and study days, transcribed the relevant sections and made notes on the remainder of the contents.

FolioViews Infobase Production Kit version 3.1 (Folio Corporation 1995) was used to facilitate data management. The data were coded according to my overall comprehension of the material. This enabled me to access data relating to particular themes and to undertake further detailed analysis and sub-categorization.

Ethical considerations

Informed consent

I wanted to be as overt about my research interests as possible. There was no reason for the study to be undertaken covertly and I would have felt deeply uncomfortable with anything other than an honest approach. I openly took notes and often walked about the ward areas with my note book in my hand. I did not often make notes during conversations as it tended to stifle the flow of talk but I did so overtly straight afterwards. For example, I would often remark – 'That's very interesting. I'd better go and write all that down before I forget it.' There were some occasions when I was privy to talk, particularly in the canteen, that participants might not have perceived as having relevance to the research, but I reasoned that having been exposed to the information it would influence my interpretation of the other data that I had and, in the interests of methodological rigour, it was better to record it. I have made special efforts to treat this material sensitively.

In setting out ethical considerations in the research outline, which was distributed to the study participants, I stated that the informed consent of all those involved in the research would be sought. This was easier in theory than in practice, however, and in actuality, the research was more or less overt depending on the circumstances. Dingwall (1980) has highlighted the moral dilemmas caused by the strategy of minimal intervention preferred by ethnographers. One particular difficulty I encountered was that the continuous throughput of different personnel on the wards meant that I encountered and observed many people during the course of the fieldwork who had little idea of my purposes. When it was appropriate I explained my research to them but on many occasions this was not possible. For example, on one occasion, when I was shadowing a junior doctor he was called to a cardiac arrest. While he involved himself in the resuscitation effort, I positioned myself unobtrusively on the periphery of the scene. One of the medical team insisted that I observed the resuscitation effort more closely, however, and ushered me towards the space he had made for me in the crowd surrounding the patient and then went on to explain the proceedings. He clearly mistook me for a medical student and, given the circumstances, it was easier to 'go with the flow' rather than enter into a detailed explanation of my true purposes.

While every effort has been taken to ensure the anonymity of field actors, by the use of pseudonyms, there are real difficulties in maintaining anonymity in the case of certain individuals whose position in the organization makes them more readily identifiable by someone with a knowledge of the field setting.

Being a nurse researching nurses

One issue that is often raised in the methodological literature (Burgess 1984) is of the relative advantages and disadvantages of researching settings with which one is familiar. Having a background in nursing had a number of advantages. First, I was well-versed in nursing and medical 'speak' and so, for the most part, I did not have to grapple with understanding a strange language. Second, knowing that I had a background in nursing meant that I was perceived by participants as someone who knew 'what it was really like', a factor that I felt, on the whole, made respondents more inclined to give candid accounts of their action. Third, in negotiating access to the wards I was able to persuade gatekeepers that as a result of my nursing experience I would know when to keep a low profile.

The methodological literature suggests that familiarity with a setting may disadvantage the researcher in that it may be difficult to recognize cultural patterns other than those things that are conventionally there to be seen. The way in which I endeavoured to deal with this was by taking detailed fieldnotes of my observations which, as I have indicated, had a behaviourist character. As Burgess (1984) has pointed out, however, the debate concerning the degree of familiarity or strangeness the sociologist may encounter in a cultural setting has been polarized in some of the literature. Situations are neither totally familiar or totally strange. As a nurse researching nursing I, like Robinson (1992), was not studying a strange tribe. Nevertheless, I had not practised as a nurse for some five years and I had never worked at Woodlands and so there were many things that were strange to me. But as a nurse studying contemporary nursing issues I could only play the naive researcher to a limited extent, and many of the interviews I carried out and the conversations I had took a form that more resembled a dialogue between two people grappling with the problems facing practitioners in the 1990s. This was particularly the case with many of the senior nurses who, because of the positions they occupied within the organization, had a special interest in the subject of my research.

Concluding comments

The selection of any research method inevitably entails a trade-off and while ethnography was the most appropriate method given my research interests it nevertheless has characteristic weaknesses. A common criticism relates to the question of research validity. Put simply, how does one know whether the participant observer has provided a totally subjective account? I have tried to address this issue in several ways. First, as I indicated at the start of the chapter, following Hammersley and Atkinson, I have endeavoured to lay the research process bare in order to allow the reader to assess the study's validity. Second, as far as limitations of space permit, I have made the data available to the reader in order that the strength of my interpretations can be judged. In the past, a problem with much ethnographic work has been the looseness of the relationship between the data and the analysis. Thirdly, as I have mentioned, fieldnotes were behaviourist or low-inference in style.

4

THE INTRA-OCCUPATIONAL DIVISION OF LABOUR

In this chapter I introduce the ward nurses and examine the ways in which they organized and negotiated their work. As we saw in Chapter 1, the discourses of professionalism and managerialism both had implications for the intra-occupational division of labour. Project 2000 was, amongst other things, an attempt to instigate profound changes to the organization of nursing practice. Founded on a philosophy of holism, it advocated a shift away from the old system of hierarchical task allocation and a reintegration of all caring work into the clinical nursing role. Under this new method of work organization, the caring division of labour is centred on a close interpersonal relationship between nurse and patient. Emphasis is also given to practitioner autonomy and accountability for patient care.

At one level certainly, 'new nursing' is a mode of practice that resonates well with the discourses of managerialism. For example, primary nursing fits with a decentralized approach to management in which ward sisters become budget holders and primary nurses are held responsible for the care they give (Bowers 1989). Moreover, there is a degree of convergence around models of devolved responsibility as exemplified by the 'named nurse' initiative, for instance. At the same time, however, other elements of managerialism appear to pull in the opposite direction to the professional view. For example, cost containment concerns have reduced and diluted the nursing work force to a level that is a long way removed from the professional vision of nursing based on a skill-mix rich in qualified staff. Moreover, the very notion of 'management' is anathema to the professional model of the autonomous practitioner engaged in a therapeutic alliance with his or her patient. In this chapter I explore the processes through which nurses at Woodlands managed these tensions.

The nurses

The ward-based nurses included ENs, RNs (staff nurses) and sisters who were at different stages in their careers, had different levels of experience and had worked on the wards for varying lengths of time. On Treetops, the nursing staff was bifurcated into two camps: 'homeguard' (Hughes *et al.* 1958) and 'newcomers'. The homeguard nurses were older and had extensive urology experience. Some of them had worked together for 14 years and the senior sister, senior staff nurse and enrolled nurse had been friends for 25 years. The newcomers were all junior staff nurses who had recently qualified and/or had worked on the ward for less than a year. Ward staff typified themselves in terms of the 'older' and 'younger' nurses, although the divisions between them actually related as much to the length of time they had worked on the ward as it did their age. There was no such segmentation on Fernlea. Only one of the staff nurses had qualified within the preceding year. The others had worked on the ward for at least 18 months and in one case for as long as nine years. A significant number of the ward nurses had worked together for between two and five years.

On both wards, students formed a distinct group within the nursing body. Not only were they unqualified, they were also transient members of the ward team. The students I encountered were all in their third year of training and therefore quite experienced. Some were undergoing the traditional apprenticeship style of pre-registration education, others were Project 2000 learners. Although, as a result of Project 2000, their contribution to service provision had been reduced, in both settings – because of their seniority – the students were included in the staffing numbers. As a group, the students had quite specific concerns: success-fully completing their studies, gaining the practical experience they felt they needed in order to function as a competent staff nurse, feeling part of the ward team and, ultimately, getting a job in the hospital once they had qualified.

Organizing nursing work at Woodlands

Although nurse managers believed that primary nursing was the optimum system for the organization of patient care, they recognized that its implementation at Woodlands was unrealistic given their staffing levels. They advocated a team nursing model that was seen as a 'stepping stone' towards the more holistic approach offered by primary nursing.[1]

Team nursing was first developed in North America in the 1950s and 1960s and is based on a differentiation of tasks among a stratified work force (Brannon 1994). In various wards throughout the Trust, team nursing was being implemented in slightly different ways according to their respective needs and resources. Treetops and Fernlea had employed a similar approach. This entailed the creation of two teams comprised of a mixture of qualified staff, support workers and students. Each team was headed by a nurse, who assumed responsibility for the management and supervision of care. Patients were allocated to a team for the duration of their hospital admission in order to promote continuity. Responsibility for the co-ordination of overall ward activity fell to the senior nurses in both settings.

Negotiating the intra-occupational division of labour on Treetops

I was first made aware of the significance of the intra-occupational division of labour by nurses' complaints about 'doing the obs', that is, the measurement and recording of patients' temperature, pulse, respirations and blood pressure. As I have argued in the introduction, influenced by Hughes' concept of dirty work (Hughes 1984), I was interested to uncover any aspects of their role nurses found morally polluting. In practical terms this meant entering the field setting with a sensitivity to those aspects of their work nurses either complained about or attempted to distance themselves from in their accounts of their practice.

Being a surgical ward, the observation of patients' vital signs was a recurrent activity on Treetops, particularly in the immediate post-operative period. Nurses bemoaned the frequency with which these activities were carried out and the attendant drudgery of the task. As the fieldwork progressed, however, it became apparent that nurses' complaints about 'doing the obs' were not a straightforward reflection of their antipathy towards the work activity itself, they were also an indicator of a wider dispute over the way in which the work was organized on the ward.

The nursing division of labour on Treetops was marked by a tension between the senior staff nurses and the two sisters – who were all members of the homeguard – and the newcomer junior nurses and students. These strains related to the work content of the two groups and its control. There was a clear division of labour on the ward between the junior and senior nursing staff. For the most part, it was the senior nurses who were in overall charge of the ward while the junior nurses led the teams. Junior nurses did mostly patient contact work – physical tending, technical tasks, caring for patients in the periods before and after surgery, and the processing of new admissions to the ward. They worked mainly in the patient bay areas and at particular times of the day their work overlapped with that of support staff. The senior nurses typically did the ward rounds, administered medications, co-ordinated ward activities, liaised with doctors, answered the telephone and undertook a disproportionate amount of administrative work – such as patient discharge planning. Their work centred on the area around the nurses' station, which was separated from the patient bays by a corridor.

The newcomer nurses and students complained that team nursing did not work well on the ward. They attributed this to a lack of support for the concept by the established nursing staff and the reluctance of senior nurses to relinquish control over the work and delegate activities traditionally ascribed a high status to junior colleagues. Doctors' rounds, drugs administration, and patient discharges should be devolved to the team leaders, it was argued. Junior nurses derided key senior members of staff for their status consciousness and portrayed them as needing to perform these activities in order to bolster their position within the ward hierarchy. Newcomer nurses also complained that the ward was 'run from the top' and that some senior nurses did not allow them the freedom to order their own work. It was felt that the senior sister found it particularly difficult to devolve responsibility to junior staff.

Senior nurses, for their part, maintained that it would be impractical to change the existing division of labour and devolve patient management activities to the team leaders, arguing that it would take too many staff away from patient care delivery. They insisted that senior staff should attend the consultants' ward rounds as they needed to have an overall view of the work in order to co-ordinate ward activity. The staffing numbers did not permit both the senior nurse *and* the team leaders to attend, they argued. Furthermore, as there were no HOs allocated to Treetops, it was the nurses who presented the patients to the consultants on the ward round and updated them on their progress. Senior nurses believed that many of the junior nurses were too inexperienced to assume this responsibility and claimed that some could be 'over-confident'.

It seemed initially that these intra-occupational strains reflected a straightforward tension between the old and the new order, that is, between the senior nurses' management version of nursing, which dominated the occupation for a large part of its history, and the 'new' professionalism of more recently trained staff. Notice in the following extracts, for example, how the junior nurses employ a contrastive rhetoric (Hargreaves 1981) in which they juxtapose patient-centred philosophies of care with the task-oriented approach of senior staff.

I don't mind doing anything if it's for the patient because that's why I'm here, I'm here for the patient not for anybody else. Obs are part of your daily work and they need doing. What I do object to is being given them to do as a task and not for the patient's benefit.

(Staff Nurse)

Once I was bed-bathing this man who was quite poorly and she (Sister) came rushing in: 'Can you go in the sluice and tie up the skip bags because we haven't got an auxiliary on this morning.' So I thought 'I can't believe this', so I said, 'Yes I'm just doing this', and she says 'No, do it now. Do it now because it's a very important job.' Well I thought 'I've got this man here laid naked on his bed half way through a bed bath and she wants me to leave him and go and do skip bags!' and like a fool I went and did it because she just made such a fuss about it.

(Staff Nurse)

On reflection, however, although the rhetoric of patient-centredness and holistic care figured prominently in the nurses' accounts, it seemed that the intra-occupational conflict was primarily concerned with the implications that the system of work had for junior nurses' job satisfaction and their sense of professional esteem, rather than a reflection of their strong commitment to primary nursing as an ideal model of nursing practice. Indeed, although the nurses subscribed to an ideology of individualized patient care, the organization of nursing work on Treetops was essentially pragmatic. It embraced elements of primary nursing, team nursing and task allocation with the precise balance of these elements being continuously modified in response to the contingencies of the work setting. These findings echo those of Savage (1995) who employed ethnographic research methods to explore nursing intimacy on two wards in the UK where different modes of patient care delivery were employed.

> One of the clearest points to emerge from discussions with nurses about organizational modes was that it cannot be assumed that the introduction of primary nursing, by itself, is evidence of a more progressive approach to nursing, or suggests a greater commitment to patient care than exists where other ways of working are employed. A similar commitment to care may be differently expressed, according to local conditions, the priorities that shape the organization of care, and the impact of either one of these upon each other.

(Savage 1995: 49)

Although most staff at Woodlands conceded that their approach to care delivery was a long way removed from the idealized primary nursing models, it was generally considered to be a realistic response to the constraints within which they practised. It was the implications that the intra-occupational division of labour had for their job satisfaction and professional identities that junior nurses struggled to accommodate. Their discontent with the organization of work on the ward centred on three themes. First, it related to the belief that work should be allocated fairly. Second, it reflected the view that the team leaders should have greater control over how they ordered their work. Third, it concerned the implications that the organization of ward work had for nurses' sense of professional competence.

A fair allocation of work

The junior nurses and students subscribed to the belief that work should be allocated 'fairly'. They claimed that senior staff were 'lazy' and would do anything that allowed them to 'sit down' while they did all the 'work', which was defined in terms of the physical and emotional labour (Hochschild 1983; James 1989; Smith 1992) involved in direct patient care. As we shall see in Chapter 6, almost without exception, nursing staff complained about the amount of paperwork they were expected to do, but rather than being grateful to those members who undertook a disproportionate share, their colleagues criticized them for their idleness. Paperwork, unlike patient work, was not seen as real work.

STAFF NURSE: *(Y)ou tend to get some staff nurses that would rather sit at the desk pushing the pen than actually doing anything.*
DA: *By doing anything?*
STAFF NURSE: *Well I mean physically doing anything.*

Both senior and newcomer junior nurses typified each other as preoccupied with paperwork and unconcerned with patient contact work. Individuals who were prepared to 'muck in' and 'pull their weight' were well-regarded.

> *I just like to work together. You just all muck in. If one's doing something and somebody needs something then you just do it. You don't say, 'Oh you're not in my team.' It doesn't happen.*
>
> (EN)

Somebody who's good to work with anyway not just a good nurse to work with but a good work mate is somebody who pulls their weight, doesn't give you the jobs that they don't want to do, who's good at their job as well.

(Student Nurse)

Lydia [HCA] describes Julie [staff nurse] as a 'mucker'. 'She really gets down to it.'

Other studies have also highlighted the importance within nursing of 'getting through the work' (Clarke 1978; Melia 1987). Clarke has argued that the language nurses use emphasizes this perspective: 'the work load', 'working hard', 'pulling your weight', 'pulling together', 'mucking in', 'like horses', 'getting through it', 'getting on with it' (Clarke 1978: 76–8). There are obvious similarities here with the nomenclature used by the nurses at Woodlands.

The nurses' accounts of their work suggest that although patient contact work is now more highly valued than it was in the past, staff found it difficult to sustain when it was performed without interruption by other kinds of work. As Strauss *et al.* (1985) point out, dirty work is a potential aspect of all work. Tasks can become so exhausting or stressful as to tip towards the non-gratifying and ultimately the dirty side of work.

It's not fair to put it [hands-on care] all on a small group of people. It can't be any good for the patients because I don't care who you are there comes a point when you think, 'Oh I've just had enough.'

(Student)

Doris [EN] said that she didn't like working with Ellen [staff nurse] because she didn't want to do anything. 'She doesn't touch a patient [...] when I leave here in the morning after working with her I'm on my knees.'

In employing the discourse of professionalism then, it would seem that the nurses were not necessarily invoking an ideal model of holistic *patient*-centred care, rather they were referring to a preferred *division of labour* in which the demands of caring work could be paced by mixing and balancing a range of activities.

I like to do a bit of everything in the day if I can.

(Student)

Writing from a psychodynamic perspective, Menzies (1963) has suggested that task allocation served an important function in protecting nurses against the anxiety of dealing with human suffering. My findings indicate that the division of labour on Treetops in which junior nurses and support staff undertook the bulk of the caring work created work strains. Nurses' vocabularies of holistic care can be seen as an attempt to manage these pressures and to negotiate for themselves a less onerous bundle of work. Indeed, some of the nurses I interviewed admitted to occasionally using paperwork in order to gain some respite from the physical and emotional labour of patient contact work.

DA: *Do we ever use the paperwork as a way of escaping from the patients?*

STAFF NURSE: *Oh yes – definitely – yes sometimes definitely yes. Sometimes you think a patient really wants to talk to you and they've been on at you all day about the same things so you say 'I've got to go and do my work now. Talk to me after because I've got quite a lot to do and I've got all these patients to write up you know' [...] I'd be lying if I said different.*

Work control

The intra-occupational tensions on Treetops also related to the nurses' efforts to control their work. A major complaint was that senior staff did not allow the team leaders to organize their work priorities.

[Y]ou can be half way through a job and they say 'Can you do this? Will you do this for me?' Rather than just giving you a list of jobs and saying 'This is what needs getting done' and then going off and getting it done because you can just prioritise it yourself rather than getting things thrown at you when you're in the middle of something else.

(Staff Nurse)

[I]f we're having teams then I think it should be up to us to say who does what. It really does get on my nerves sometimes when Sister will say 'Now will you make sure you do that', and it might not even be for your team. 'Will you make sure that man has a drink every hour' or 'You'll do that won't you?', and it really does rile me.

(Staff Nurse)

The sister herself spoke of the difficulties she had experienced in 'letting go'.

I must say I did find it hard to withdraw – if you know what I mean – from giving the hands-on experience. I was trying to do too much.

(Senior Sister)

The junior nurses employed various strategies in avoiding what they considered to be illegitimate control of their work.

John [student] [...] had a trolley in the bay and some of the patient's kardexes. I said, 'What are you doing?' 'John' replied, 'filing' [...] Then he said, 'Damn I need a divider', he looked out of the bay and said, 'Where's Sister? Can I go and get this without being set off to do another job?'

I found Brenda [staff nurse], the student and the auxiliary behind the curtains. The student and the auxiliary were giving Mr Edwards a wash. I said that I had come to see if I could help but that I could see there were probably enough of them there already. Brenda said that she wasn't involved, she was just hiding from the senior sister so that she could not give her any more jobs to do. 'I've done fifty thousand different jobs already this morning,' she said. The student nurse quipped 'Only 50 thousand? You're lucky.' The auxiliary observed that she must have had an easy morning. They all laughed. 'Actually,' Brenda said, 'I'm not skiving, I have two men on the toilet.'

It was the senior nurses, however, who had an overview of the shifting priorities on the ward as a whole, whereas team leaders were more narrowly focused on the needs of their specific patients and, as I described in Chapter 3, the pace of work on Treetops could change dramatically. Moreover, because of the need to adhere to operating theatre schedules, nursing work on Treetops was more tightly locked into external organizational timetables than it was on Fernlea ward. Senior nurses were also very conscious of the relative inexperience of the newcomer junior nursing staff and had a strong sense of their own responsibility for the care of all patients on the ward.

[A]ll right an RGN's responsible for her own actions but it is my ward.

(Senior Sister)

Knowing the patient

In addition to issues of fairness and work control, the struggles over the organization of nursing work also centred on the business of 'knowing the patient' and its relationship to nurses' sense of professional expertise. The 'new nursing' discourse emphasizes the importance of the nurse–patient relationship and its therapeutic potential (Ersser 1997). A corollary of this professional vision is that 'knowing the patient' becomes an important marker of a practitioner's competence. For the nurses at Woodlands 'knowing the patient' related to having up-to-date knowledge of the patient's progress and their relevant social circumstances. It did not seem to imply the level of intimacy suggested by some interpretations of nursing's 'therapeutic gaze' (see, for example, May 1992). Indeed, in clear resonances with Savage's (1995) findings, some of the study participants expressed discomfort at the types of information required by the nursing assessment pro forma. Nevertheless, despite this tempering of the professional vision, for the nurses at Woodlands to 'know' all aspects of care relating to one's patient was to accomplish a convincing professional performance.

Because much of nursing work is invisible, the ritual of nursing handover (Wolf 1988, 2000) is a key forum in which, *inter alia,* nurses' professional skills can be demonstrated (see also Parker *et al.* 1992). For neophyte nurses, handover is an important arena in which they can learn what it means to be a good nurse (Wolf 1988). Handover took place three times a day. It involved an oral summary and update on each patient's progress by the nurses who had been caring for them to the staff about to commence the next shift. The junior nurses complained that because of the way in which the work was organized on the ward there would often be key aspects of their patient's care that they were unaware of.

> *[W]hen it comes to handover there's all these patients that have been admitted and you haven't admitted one of these. [...] And you're reading through slowly and you're going 'Er er er', you just can't flow freely. If you've been through it with them then you can go through the main problems, everything.*
>
> (Staff Nurse)

The junior nurses complained that senior nurses always 'interjected' when they were trying to present their patients and this was a source of frustration and tension.

As the nurses assembled for handover, Geraldine (staff nurse) jokingly remarked to the senior sister that there 'were not to be any interjections'. Sister said that the issue of interjections had come up on the student evaluation, but she wanted to stress that it was important that all the information was passed on and thus many of the interjections were necessary.

You're doing handover for your team and you come to a patient and you think, 'Oh I haven't even seen this patient', and that's when it breaks down [...] Then you get this friction you know because you think she's butting in.

(Staff Nurse)

Drawing on Kelly and May (1982), May (1992) has observed that nurses categorize medical staff as 'good' or 'bad' according to whether they support their professional performance by passing information on to them or not. May argues that 'bad' doctors were those who disrupted the flow of information and made it difficult for nurses to 'know the patient'. Given the reality of hospital nursing, however, there is a sense in which these sorts of difficulties are inevitable. The rhetoric of 'knowing the patient' is based on the professional ideal of a close inter-personal relationship between client and carer, but in most hospitals wards care has to be provided simultaneously to a number of different patients in a multi-professional setting bounded by an uncertain work environment. In coping with these tensions nurses had adopted a pragmatic model of work organization and, as a consequence, 'knowing the patient' was always a collective rather than an individual accomplishment. Nevertheless, the disproportionate amount of patient management undertaken by senior staff on Treetops made it even more difficult for nurses to acquire a full knowledge of these aspects of patient care, compounding a contradictory state of affairs that already threatened their sense of professional identity.

Fernlea ward – a comparison

On Fernlea, ward activities were ordered very differently. Nursing work was organized in a non-hierarchical manner. Senior nurses referred to themselves as 'co-ordinating' the ward, whereas on Treetops they described themselves as being 'in-charge' of it. With the exception of drug administration, responsibility for all aspects of patient care-management was devolved to the team leaders who also had greater control over their work. The intra-occupational division of labour was less fraught with the tensions of the surgical setting. Like the urology ward, the nurses on Fernlea employed a pragmatic mode of work organization that combined elements of primary nursing, team nursing and task allocation. The fair allocation of work was also clearly considered to be important, but student nurses spoke highly of their experiences and junior nurses believed that, for the most part, work was equitably distributed.

> *I think we're quite sort of fair on the ward to be honest.*
> (Staff Nurse)

The poverty of the co-ordinator role

Although junior staff were mainly happy with the content of their work, the extent of devolution on Fernlea meant that the ward co-ordinator role was problematic and key senior staff on the ward were deeply dissatisfied.

> *It's a bit of a nondescript role really. You're there for help if they need any help. It's a bit of a funny role really.*
> (Junior Sister)

> *I don't think the co-ordinator's role is very well defined on here. All they seem to do is drugs and that's not really as it should be I don't think.*
> (Staff Nurse)

Several of the senior nurses referred to their efforts to reintegrate devolved activities into their work.

> *If they're very busy I'll do the ward round for them and pass that on – I try and poach little bits back.*
> (Junior Sister)

> *You know – typical scenario – I'm in the bathroom and they'll come in and go 'What are you doing in here?' You know 'Come out!', and I'm like 'No I want to!' 'You shouldn't be bathing you've got other things to do' and I think 'No I'll do the other things later I'd just like to bath this person', and sometimes I really have to stand my ground. I know they're only thinking of me because I have got the paperwork and boring jobs to do that they think I shouldn't be doing that. You know it's like if somebody wants turning I'll say 'Would you like to give me a hand to turn somebody?', and they'll say 'No I'll do it, I'll do it. You're all right.' You know and I'm thinking 'No I want to do*

it!' – you know – 'I'm here this is what I'm here for and this is what I'm paid for as well'. I'm not paid to sit at a desk and do paperwork.

(Staff Nurse)

Sometimes the co-ordinators' attempts to carve out a more rewarding role created tension:

JUNIOR SISTER: Sarah can I put you as 'named nurse'?
STAFF NURSE: It's all right, I'll do it.
JUNIOR SISTER: [raises voice slightly] Can I do *anything*?!
STAFF NURSE: Sorry.

Work control

Control of nursing work was again problematic but the issues on Fernlea were rather different from those on the surgical ward. As on Treetops, the team leaders expected to be left to organize their own work and disliked intrusions. One of the ward co-ordinators acknowledged the need to be sensitive to the team leaders' need for independence.

I asked Lorraine what the co-ordinator did apart from the drugs.

LORRAINE: Co-ordinate! And poke this [points to nose] in. I do it subtly and they don't know I'm doing it but some of them haven't been qualified that long and they need a bit of guidance. I have to be careful how I do it. I ask questions as reminders. I might say 'Is Mr so-and-so ready for theatre yet?' Meaning 'Get Mr so-and-so ready for theatre.'

Despite their wish for autonomy, there was a general agreement amongst the junior nurses that the senior sister had taken devolution too far and did not take responsibility for the ward as a whole. They criticized her for spending too much time away from the ward doing office work. In contrast to the situation on Treetops ward where the participation of certain nursing staff in drug administration was seen as evidence of their status consciousness, on Fernlea the lack of involvement of the senior sister in medication rounds was regarded as a symbol of her withdrawal from the clinical setting. Staff were left feeling vulnerable and insecure and this placed an intolerable burden on the junior sister who was frequently contacted at home by nurses seeking reassurance that

71

they had taken the right course of action. At the time of the study these pressures were beginning to take their toll.

I got into quite a state about it and quite upset [...] I was getting really stressed out there, and if anything goes off the girls come to me with problems because I think they feel that Sister won't sort them. So I get 99 per cent of all the problems and if there's anything now coming through complaints-wise – they all come to me to be sorted so I feel as if [...] I don't know what to do next.[...] It's a terrible situation and I get quite upset when I think about it [...]. I feel as though I've taken over totally and I don't want to do it any more [Tape recorder was turned off].

(Junior Sister)

Knowing the patient

There were also intra-occupational tensions on Fernlea relating to 'knowing the patient' but again these were of a rather different kind from those I have described on Treetops. Despite their devolution of care management to the team leaders, all the senior nurses responsible for co-ordinating ward activity strongly believed that they should continue to have a knowledge of the details of medical and nursing care for all patients on the ward. They complained that often the team leaders did not communicate the information they needed back to them, which left them feeling exposed in a number of ways.

I'm always the co-ordinator if I'm on and I feel lost sometimes. If there are some juniors and students on they feed back to me a bit so I know more what's going on but some of the others they're quite protective of their team and they like to sort out their own problems. So a consultant might come on to the ward and expect me to have the answers and I don't know what's going on. So I have to say 'This nurse has been looking after him.'

(Senior Sister)

It was felt that reporting back to colleagues after ward rounds had unfortunately stopped. Please could this practice be recommenced as it can be both frustrating and embarrassing at times for colleagues who are expected to know what is occurring on the ward.

(Document – minutes from ward meeting)

Also the results of each ward round should be entered into the nursing kardex. May we also remind staff that sisters need to be kept aware that although not in a 'team' we are accountable for your actions and often relatives do approach us for information.

(Document – minutes from ward meeting)

These extracts indicate that at one level certainly, the pressure for senior nurses to 'know the patient(s)' appeared to come from the perception that relatives and doctors expected them to have all the necessary information at hand. In the past, it was the ward sister or charge nurse who was the repository of knowledge on the ward and all nursing decisions were filtered through them and, as Abbott (1988) has suggested, public perceptions of occupational jurisdiction can last for years after change has occurred. These tensions cannot be explained solely in terms of an historical legacy however. Notice also, how the extracts contain references to senior nurses' sense of clinical accountability and their discomfiture when they do not have immediate access to patient information. Arguably, a further factor contributing to these strains are the contradictory prescriptions for practice contained in the discourses of professionalism and managerialism that placed the ward co-ordinators in a double-bind.

Although professional models of nursing advocate the devolution of clinical responsibility to individual practitioners they also promote intimate knowledge of the patient as the apotheosis of professional practice. This is a vision of the 'good nurse' that senior staff are clearly not immune to even if the daily reality of their work is only remotely related to this private-practice model. Moreover, both management and professional discourses emphasize practitioner accountability and risk management. The upshot of these dual pressures was that for senior nurses, as for their junior colleagues, 'knowing the patient' was also oriented to as a master professional trait. To not 'know', threatened their sense of professional competence in fundamental ways.

Gina [junior sister] is presenting a patient. There is a pause in her delivery.
STAFF NURSE: Can I just add her blood pressure's up.
GINA: Wait a minute. I've not finished. I'm just looking for another section.

Understanding the strains?

Although the intra-occupational tension on the wards was of different kinds, at root was a common problem of the division of labour between the team leaders and the nurses with overall responsibility for running the ward. On Treetops, senior staff were reluctant to let go of the traditional functions of the ward sister to the dissatisfaction of junior nursing staff. On Fernlea, where senior nurses had managed to devolve most aspects of patient management, they had been left with a vacuum they had been unable to fill to their satisfaction, and, in the case of one senior nurse, responsibility had been devolved so far that junior staff were left feeling vulnerable.

At one level, the boundary disputes on the ward can be understood as a reflection of the change process and the need for staff to adjust to the role-realignment occasioned by the ideologies of Project 2000. In mapping out the pre-conditions necessary for 'new nursing', Beardshaw and Robinson (1990) underline the need for the ward sister's role to shift from involvement in supervising and administering to an emphasis on clinical consultancy, staff support, ward management and planning and co-ordination of research and education. Beardshaw and Robinson concede that research into the way that ward sisters work makes it clear that few are currently trained and equipped to function in this way, nor are they enabled to by higher level management. At Woodlands, certainly, changes to the ward sister's role were occurring largely by default. No provision had been made to help ward sisters prepare for these shifts in the boundaries of their work. Indeed, similar scenarios were being played out throughout the organization. Yet despite the lack of organizational support for the change process, senior managers appeared to attribute these tensions to the inability of the ward sisters to accommodate change.

> *I think the other thing has been the change in the actual sister's role. It has become more management orientated, there is very little opportunity for clinical input and as a result of that sisters felt extremely threatened. Once upon a time, in my time, as a sister, you were the person that everybody was homing in to and you were expected to know every little detail for your patient, from the general issues to blood values, and because that was the custom that is still the perception some of the sisters still have of their role. And it has been very, very hard in having the team organization within the nursing structure to let go. They were feeling awfully threatened and yet they were*

feeling awfully under duress for the volume of work that was circulating around. It was a struggle to achieve the transition and some had more difficulty than others to come to terms with the change. And some have been able to develop more than others and exercise the delegation of duties to make the best possible use of the F grade or even the Es and every member of the team. But it all depends on individuals and sometimes people see it as a threat.

(CMT – Nurse Manager)

These findings do appear to be supported elsewhere in the literature. For example, Webb and Pontin (1996), researching the implementation of primary nursing on four wards, found that the 'ward co-ordinator' and 'deputy ward co-ordinator' maintained that they had insufficient information about direct clinical care issues and this left them feeling vulnerable to accusations of negligence. Other studies have also described the ward manager's role under the primary nursing system as fraught with contradictions (Titchen and Binnie 1993; Willmott 1998). These authors criticize Trust management for inadequate consultation processes and failure to fully prepare staff. The logical conclusion of this line of argument, however, is that had change been strategically managed then these difficulties could have been avoided. I suggest this is an over-simplification of the problem. To be fully comprehended these issues have to be considered in terms of the deeply entrenched strains between professional and management discourses.

At a far more fundamental level, the intra-occupational tensions on the wards were a product of the difficulties practitioners faced in reconciling professional models of care with the workplace reality of hospital nursing. Nurses are subject to conflicting and ambiguous ideologies. The professional rhetoric of 'new nursing' emphasizes their status as autonomous practitioners but as employees in a managed organization nurses are expected to render obedience to superiors and conform to formal rules and regulations. Project 2000 left traditional nursing structures firmly intact. Primary nursing models recommend that ward sisters devolve patient management to clinical staff and yet, at the same time, professional discourses also emphasize the nurse–patient relationship as the foundation and essence of nursing practice and new managerialism has heralded an increased concern for risk management, individual responsibility and accountability. Professional and management discourses both encourage the withdrawal of the ward sister from direct clinical care work, and yet at Woodlands certainly, ward sisters were included in the ward staffing numbers. 'New nursing' emphasizes the centrality of the nurse–patient relationship, but nurses work with multiple assignments in a turbulent (Melia 1979) work environment.

The nurses on both wards appeared to have accommodated themselves to certain of these tensions. They employed a pragmatic rather than a purist approach to the organization of ward work and were realistic about what was achievable within existing staffing levels. Yet other aspects of these tensions appeared less easy for the nurses to reconcile. I have suggested that for nurses the most intolerable strains were those that profoundly affected their sense of professional identity. First, there was the discontinuity between the rhetoric of clinical autonomy and the workplace reality of occupational hierarchy that generated stress in relation to the content and control of nursing work. Second, there was the disjuncture between the private-practice model of professionalism based on an intimate one-to-one relationship with the patient and the multiple assignments that characterize real life hospital nursing, which was reflected in the tensions surrounding the division of caring work and 'knowing the patient'.

As Hart (1989) has observed, because nursing work relies on staff working together and because work is allocated in a personalized manner, it becomes all too easy for nurses to blame one another for the contradictions in the system. The intra-occupational division of labour on both wards was accomplished by dint of a great deal of negotiative effort and, for the most part, the nurses managed to contain these interpersonal strains. There remained an undercurrent, however, which regularly surfaced in backstage regions such as the canteen, and occasionally on the ward itself. During their interviews some members of staff broke down and wept such was their frustration with work colleagues. It seemed that for ward staff managing the tensions in the system was a fundamental work skill.

5

THE NURSE–
SUPPORT WORKER
BOUNDARY

Unqualified support staff have long been the proverbial thorn in the side of those who subscribe to a professional vision of nursing. Despite a deep-rooted desire for an all-qualified work force by certain segments of the occupation, nursing has thus far failed to secure jurisdictional closure (Witz 1988). Owing to demographic and economic pressures (paid) nursing care has always been provided by a mixture of qualified and unqualified staff, and, contrary to much nursing rhetoric, it is students and auxiliaries who have undertaken most of the direct physical tending of patients.

I described in Chapter 1 how government acceptance of the Project 2000 reforms hinged on its proponents agreeing to the introduction of a new category of support worker: the health care assistant (HCA). This was a trade-off that was to compromise the professional vision of nursing in important, although often unarticulated, ways. It meant that nurses were exposed to contradictory discourses: on the one hand, a professional discourse which emphasized the need to *reclaim* 'hands-on' care as a legitimate aspect of the nursing role and, on the other, a management discourse that pointed to the need for practitioners to *relinquish* further 'technical' aspects of nursing work to HCAs. Moreover, the holistic model of nursing on which the Project 2000 reforms was based, was predicated on the assumption of a richly skilled work force, and yet there is evidence to suggest that the formula devised by the Department of Health for the calculation of replacement staff led to significant staff shortages at ward level (Elkan *et al.* 1994). These developments raised important jurisdictional dilemmas for nurses but it was left to the local level to decide how care was to be provided within the resources available.

In this chapter I explore the ways in which nurses at Woodlands were responding to these tensions and examine how the nurse–support worker boundary was being produced in a number of arenas throughout the hospital. Although there has been considerable research interest in the division of labour between nurses and support workers in recent years, this work has either been underpinned by a task-oriented approach – in which judgements are made about what does (or does not) constitute a legitimate deployment of registered nursing skills – or a people-oriented approach in which nurses and/or support workers' opinions of their respective roles and responsibilities are sought. To the best of my knowledge there is little empirical research that focuses on the *processes* via which the nurse–support worker boundary is managed in daily practice.

The nurse–support worker boundary at Woodlands: an overview

Although the introduction of HCAs into the health services division of labour was well underway at the time of the study, conversations with senior staff suggested that there has been some local variation in the role's implementation. For example, one hospital in the region had made all its existing auxiliaries HCAs overnight, simply by changing their job title. At Woodlands, however, the HCA and the auxiliary were formally distinct roles. The HCAs had a different title and job description and, although they wore the same dresses as auxiliaries, they were provided with coloured belts that signified difference. Moreover, unlike the auxiliaries, who developed their skills on the job, the HCAs undertook classroom-based learning. A 25-day training course was devised and taught by Greta, the nurse manager with responsibility for the implementation of Project 2000. At the end of the course, HCAs were given 'log sheets' on which ward nurses had to indicate competence in specific areas of practice. In addition to the 'in-house' training, HCAs also had the opportunity to undertake an NVQ at level two but this was not compulsory. Indeed, the planned linkage of the HCA role with the NVQ framework appeared, in practice, to be a rather loose coupling. NVQs at Woodlands predated the introduction of HCAs and had been originally implemented as a 'feel good' factor. Senior nurses assumed that it would be the auxiliaries who had taken NVQs who would become the new HCAs. In practice not all of them did and the result was a discontinuity between the credentials and occupational status of many support staff.

Officially, the HCA role was wider than that of the traditional auxiliary. It embraced certain technical procedures such as measuring and recording temperature, pulse and blood pressure, collecting blood from the blood bank, taking patients to theatre, and the removal of intravenous (IV) cannulae, which were previously the remit of qualified nurses. At the time of the research, however, the work of HCAs and auxiliaries was barely distinguishable. At one level, this reflected the newness of the role: many of the HCAs were still undergoing training and, therefore, practising in a restricted capacity. This said, even the role of *experienced* HCAs was little different from that of the auxiliaries. On Fernlea, the only additional activities the HCA undertook was the measurement and recording of patients' vital signs and the removal of intravenous cannulae. On Treetops, it was the informally extended practice of the auxiliaries that accounted for the blurring of the support worker roles. Historically, Woodlands had experienced difficulties in recruiting qualified nursing staff and, owing to pressures of work, auxiliaries had been entrusted to undertake activities outside their official jurisdiction. Two of the auxiliaries on Treetops had over 10 years, experience on the ward and during this time had extended their role to embrace much of the 'little bit extra on top' that supposedly distinguished the HCAs from the auxiliaries. Because of the degree of overlap between the two roles I focused my observations on nurses' management of the support worker in general, rather than concentrating specifically on the HCAs, as was my original intention.

Accomplishing the limits of the support worker role: the 'boundary-work' of nurse managers

I am going to begin my examination of the empirical material with an analysis of the processes through which nurse managers charged, *inter alia,* with the implementation of the HCA role, negotiated role realignment. In taking the management arena as the starting point for my discussion, my aim is to provide the reader with a sense of the local organizational policy against which negotiation of the nursing–support worker boundary at ward level was situated. As a site where occupational jurisdictions are claimed and sustained, the management arena has been hitherto neglected in interactionist studies of hospital settings. The sociological eye has focused primarily on the ways in which staff in the clinical domain negotiate their occupational roles, and the formal organizational plan is typically treated as a 'background' against which the daily constitution of work boundaries takes place. Yet, as proponents of the negotiated order perspective have pointed out, the formal organizational structure is itself a negotiated order, even if it becomes more-or-less stable at particular points in time and/or for specific analytic purposes.

Nurse managers at Woodlands accepted the need for better trained support staff to compensate for the loss of student nurses' service contribution following the introduction of Project 2000. They felt that a skilled support worker would provide for a flexible division of labour on the wards and help to avoid the fragmentation of care that Project 2000 and its associated ideology was designed to overcome. They were also adamant, however, that the parameters of the HCA role should be under the control of nurses, both in formal policy and in local practice.

In this section I shall be considering the demarcatory practices nurse managers employed in their attempts to retain control over the scope of support workers' jurisdiction. I suggest that these strategies may be considered as examples of 'boundary-work'. The concept is Gieryn's (1983, 1999) and he developed it to refer to scientists' attempts to create a favourable public image for the discipline by contrasting it to non-scientific or technical activities. Gieryn argues that as intellectual debates about the boundaries of science continue, demarcation is routinely accomplished in everyday settings. As Gieryn points out, demarcation is more than an analytic problem: scientists have access to considerable material and professional opportunities that are not available to non-scientists and hence, the interactional work that is done in the social production of occupational boundaries has to be understood as a micropolitical process. Gieryn's analysis centres on 'public science', that is, the kinds of claims that are made for science in public and political arenas. As Abbott (1988) has observed (see Chapter 2), however, similar kinds of political processes can also be seen in play in the workplace, where the accomplishment of occupational jurisdiction or the doing of demarcation is a routine feature of everyday practice.

Taking control

It was nurse managers who, in consultation with the ward sisters, had defined the official limits of the HCA role. A list of activities that HCAs were permitted to undertake had been formulated and this acted as an important textual marker of the scope of HCA practice. The extent to which HCAs worked within these formally-defined boundaries was to be further determined by staff at the point of service delivery according to the requirements of the ward and the exigencies of the work. This is how Greta, the nurse manager responsible for the implementation of Project 2000, described HCA jurisdiction on an in-service training day.

[Y]ou are working in very different areas and your areas have very different needs of you and those needs will vary from time to time and I can't go along and say to you, 'You will be doing this, this, this and this.' All I can do is say to you, 'As an organization [...] we have things that have been agreed for you to actually start to undertake.'

(HCA training day – Tape)

This is a very powerful strategy for defending nursing's jurisdictional boundaries because it denies HCAs a clearly defined domain of practice. The key word for nurse managers was that the role of the HCA was to *assist* qualified staff. Thus, officially at least, the role of the HCAs was what the nurse decides that it is, on a given occasion.

Another way in which the nurse managers attempted to do demarcation was by exerting control over the education and training of HCAs. Although there was no compulsion for the HCAs at Woodlands to gain NVQ qualifications, all had to undertake the 25-day training programme provided in-house. This gave nurse managers some control over HCAs' knowledge base and also created an opportunity to undertake boundary work of other kinds. This was important because, despite this careful policing of boundaries, the nurse managers were well aware that work pressures presented a powerful countervailing force at ward-level. Training days were used as an opportunity to counteract these tendencies towards dilution and to shore up occupational frontiers.

Cautionary tales

The nurse manager responsible for HCA training had a stock of 'atrocity' (Dingwall 1977b), or 'horror' stories (Bosk 1979) that highlighted the dangers of dilution. A narrative genre that figures prominently in the medical literature, these, are tales of dramatic or shocking events that may take on a legendary or apocryphal status in the oral culture of an occupational group (Bosk 1979; Atkinson 1992). Atrocity stories have been variously analysed as mechanisms for the transmission of an occupational culture (Dingwall 1977b; Turner 1986; Atkinson 1992), moral parables that remind doctors that medicine is a serious business (Bosk 1979), vehicles for communicating shared difficulties (Dingwall 1977b; Bosk 1979; Turner 1986; Finlay *et al.* 1990), resolvers of ambiguities over occupational frontiers (Dingwall 1977b), facilitators of occupational rites of passage (Myers 1979; Hafferty 1988), relievers of anxiety and tension (Dingwall 1977b; Bosk 1979) and communicators of guilt (Bosk 1979). At Woodlands, the nurse manager employed the stories on training days for both qualified staff and HCAs as moral parables or cautionary tales in order to underline the importance of circumspection in the management of the nurse–support worker boundary.

I only went up a couple of weeks ago to work with a health care assistant and we did a bed-bath, and she hadn't really very much knowledge of this patient, and the bed-bath went on and

I just sort of followed her lead if you like because I was there in a teaching capacity but also as an observer – and the one aspect that didn't get considered was the lady's IVI. She was a bit confused this lady, had a wad of bandages on her hand of the IVI site and the HCA hadn't actually considered removing that because she said she didn't think it was her job. Fair comment. But what had happened was that nobody had thought it was their job and when we actually unravelled it – her fingers were all bent, they were so sweaty that it was like cheese, and she actually had a very tiny pressure sore development underneath her cannula site and her nails were digging in the palm of her hand, which you know, wasn't right. It wasn't quality care. But the HCA had been told that it wasn't part of her job, yet it wasn't being picked up by anybody else.

(Greta – Nurse Manager)

GRETA: I still get phone calls now saying – I had one not too many weeks ago – 'What else can the health care assistant do' and I said 'Well what are they doing?' Thinking 'I don't really want to know'. So she proceeded to tell me – this is a ward manager – proceeded to tell me this, that and the other and she said 'In fact they do everything.' So I thought 'Ah ha! So what is the registered nurse then doing?'

(HCA training day – Tape)

As we will see, these stories did have some substance: work pressures could lead to HCAs working with minimal supervision or undertaking work for which they were not trained.

Authoring the landscape

Nurse managers used the training days as an opportunity to counteract the strain towards dilution and to shore up occupational frontiers. These were 'orchestrated encounters' (Dingwall 1980) that enabled them to 'author' the organization (Shotter 1993) by formulating the 'landscape' of enabling-constraints (Giddens 1979; cited by Shotter 1993: 149) and moral positions relevant to HCAs. One of the ways in which they did this was to emphasize the possible legal implications of HCAs crossing the legitimate limits of their jurisdiction.

NURSE MANAGER [GRETA]: Now it's very easy for me to stand here and say 'You don't do this, you do that, you do the

82

other', very easy. But what I'm saying is: 'This organization will not support you if you go ahead and do these sorts of things.'

(HCA training day – Tape)

Additionally, in-service training for qualified nurses underlined their professional accountability for HCA practice. At the time of the research, concern with litigation and risk management was strong at all levels of the organization. Appealing to the legal arena was a powerful resource on which senior nurses could draw in encouraging staff to police the parameters of their practice in the face of contrary pressures from the ward.

Considerable effort also went into differentiating the role of qualified nurses from that of support staff. Indeed, an entire day on the HCA training programme was devoted to exploring the role of the registered nurse and making nursing knowledge visible. Although the HCAs questioned its relevance, from the perspective of nurse managers it was an important piece of boundary-work. The following extract is a typical example of the kinds of rhetorical devices employed on the HCA training days.

NURSE MANAGER [GRETA]: Right – you are there to *assist* the registered nurse. You're not there to do the registered nurse's job. You're there to *assist* [...] You will not be involved in assessing patients [...] You are there to *assist* in the implementation of care. Assessing patients can be anything from admitting a patient to doing a bed-bath and looking at them. As a registered nurse I can assess the situation there and then. It doesn't matter if it's the beginning of the patient's stay the middle, or the end. I am assessing all the time because that's what I have been trained to do. If you're in a position to assess then you're in the wrong position. Just let us take the TPR [temperature, pulse, and respirations] situation [...] from a registered nurse's point of view there is more to doing a pulse than just counting. I've got to know the rate, the rhythm, the depth of that pulse. By me putting my hands on that patient I am assessing that patient. I'm assessing all those different things there. If that's what is required then the registered nurse should be going in there and doing that, but if all that is required is a number then I don't see a problem with you getting in there. Assessment is a very fine line and it makes it very difficult to explain to you what you can and can't do.

(HCA training day – Tape)

There are a number of interesting features in this extract. It begins with an attempt to differentiate the support worker contribution from that of qualified staff. Notice the emphasis that is given to the role of HCAs as assistants to the registered nurse and the explicit statement that they will not be doing nursing work, which, in this instance, is formulated in terms of 'assessment'. The senior nurse goes on to underline the indeterminacy of nursing skills: '[a]ssessment is a very fine line and it makes it very difficult to explain to you what you can and can't do' which she contrasts with the narrow technical role of support staff: 'if all that is needed is a number'. As Hughes (1984), Jamous and Peloille (1970) and Abbott (1988) have pointed out, the nature of an activity is not fixed and in the context of jurisdictional battles the definition and meaning of task areas can become the subject of intense conflict. According to Jamous and Peloille (1970), the key to this is the indetermination/technicality ratio. This refers to the part played in the production process by skills that can be mastered and communicated in the form of rules in proportion to those skills that, in a given historical context, are attributed to the individual talents of producers. They argue that the indeterminate portions of a task area provide a more enduring basis for the maintenance of exclusive jurisdictional control because of their inaccessibility to the uninitiated. Professional work always contains an important margin of indetermination. Jamous and Peloille (1970) suggest that one of the ways in which a profession can defend its occupational boundaries when task areas are being taken over by other competing groups is to reduce the role of their competitors to that of 'technicians' or operatives. I suggest that this extract is a micropolitical example of precisely these kinds of processes. HCAs are rhetorically produced as making a mechanistic contribution to care compared with the sophisticated complexity of nursing practice. In fact 'assessment' is so indeterminate, that there can be no hard and fast rules as to what the HCA can or cannot do – this decision rests with the qualified member of staff.

In these diverse ways, then, nurse managers at Woodlands were involved in considerable negotiative activity in their efforts to establish jurisdictional control over support workers and differentiate the contributions of qualified and unqualified staff to the caring process. The situation on the wards, however, was rather different. Here emphasis was given to the ward team rather than divisions and differences between qualified and unqualified staff. As Zerubavel (1979) observes, co-presence is an important source of social solidarity and can be so strong as to outweigh loyalty to one's own occupational group. Moreover, the ways in which caring work was organized led to the routine blurring of the formal division of labour between nurses and support workers.

Accomplishing the nurse–support worker boundary on the wards

At the heart of the policy debates about the nurse–support worker boundary are two questions: what work should the nurse be doing and, what work should the support worker be doing? Although the subject of intense debate, these issues were left largely unanswered when Project 2000 was implemented. Nurse managers at Woodlands had expended considerable energy in addressing the latter question but appeared to give little explicit attention to the former. Rather, once the limits of support-worker jurisdiction were enshrined in local policy, it was left to ward-level staff to negotiate the content of their work within the resources available to them. In this section I use these linked questions to structure my examination of the ways in which the nurse–support worker boundary was socially produced on the wards at Woodlands.

What should the nurse be doing?

Non-nursing duties?

A central concern in the skill-mix literature is the performance of so-called 'non-nursing' duties by qualified nursing staff. Ball and Goldstone (1987) conclude that between 18 and 28 per cent of nursing time is spent on tasks that could be more suitably carried out by support staff. Leaving aside for one moment the thorny issue of what constitutes a skilled activity, it is clear that studies of this kind provide powerful ammunition for health service managers concerned with restricting nursing budgets. They provide few insights, however, into the context in which ward work is carried out and, by fragmenting work into a series of tasks rather than examining the process, they gloss over the complex ways in which patient care is organized on hospital wards.

Nurses occupy a unique place within the hospital division of labour; no other occupational group maintains 24-hour contact with patients, 365 days a year. As Davies (1995) points out, however, one of the dilemmas for the nurse in 'being there' is that s/he is not going to bother unduly with demarcation issues. At Woodlands, like any other hospital, the temporal and spatial organization of work led nurses to undertake a range of mundane activities that fell outside their formal jurisdiction – such as clerical work and portering. Although nurses performed these tasks when nobody else was available, their comments and remarks suggested that they regarded such work as illegitimate. In Hughes' (1984) terms, this was 'dirty work'. They undertook other types of 'mundane' work, however, which was handled rather differently, intertwined as it was with the process of care.

On both wards nurses regularly performed activities that an external observer might consider unskilled and easily carried out by support staff. Often the reasons for this were pragmatic. Patients' washes, meal times, observations and drug administration, formed a basic temporal structure for the delivery of patient care but within these daily routines much of the work was unpredictable. Staff were continuously readjusting their priorities in order to manage the routine and contingent aspects of their work. In the course of their everyday activities nurses undertook relatively unskilled work simply because they happened to be there at the time: the costs involved in allocating the work to somebody else frequently outweighed any advantages of delegation.

> If you happen to be there and the patient needs something then you do it for them however expensive you might be.
>
> (Sister)

> *If I'm passing and a patient wants to go to the toilet and he says 'I can't wait' then I'll take him to the toilet. I don't look round for somebody to take him. I'll do it.*
>
> (Senior Nurse)

Nurses who incurred the costs of delegation rather than undertaking low status work themselves were regarded with derision.

Most staff on both wards were critical of status consciousness and this created a particular sensitivity towards the handling of work that was literally unclean. Whereas other mundane tasks, such as making a bed, could be legitimately delegated if the nurse had other work priorities, physically dirty work tended to be managed according to the principle of 'whoever finds it, deals with it'.

DA: *If somebody found it [a soiled bed] and asked you to clear it up how would you feel about that?*
STUDENT: *I'd think well why can't you do it? And if they couldn't give me a good excuse then I'd be pissed off.*

> *I accept it if you find it and I accept it if people are busy and – say they're going round on a round for example and somebody finds somebody in a mess and then they say, 'Would you mind clearing so-and-so up?' – the times I don't like it is when somebody finds it and you know that they've got time to deal with the situation but they just pass it on.*
>
> (Auxiliary)

As Hughes (1984) has suggested, a task that is dirty can be tolerated when it is part of a good role, a role that is full of rewards to one's self. Staff accepted physically dirty work when it could be interpreted as an act of caring. When unclean work was delegated without good reason, however, it became a clear marker of the moral division of labour on the ward and was regarded as illegitimate. As we saw in Chapter 4, key members of the senior nursing staff on Treetops ward were perceived by their colleagues to be status conscious and to allocate work in a way that reflected the ward hierarchy. This was an important source of intra-occupational tension. It would seem that by demonstrating their preparedness to 'get their hands mucky' nurses were investing in their working relationships.

'Low-skilled' work activities were incorporated into nursing jurisdiction in other ways. Nurses often undertook a mundane task in order to carry out another (more complex) activity. I have called this *strategic multi-tasking*. A typical example was the use of a routine activity in order to frame an interactional encounter with patients or their families. One of the difficulties nurses faced was how to put themselves in a position to build relationships with patients in a context that was socially comfortable for both.

> *[J]ust to go round each patient, sit by them and chat to them all, it can put them on edge. If it's new staff and you can go in and do something and take the emphasis off that and see what's happening to them, they feel a little bit more relaxed. Rather than you sitting there and drilling them and seeing how they are. You know 'Open up to me. Tell me all your problems.'*
>
> (Staff Nurse)

> *I would go and make a few beds but not 'make the beds'. I would do it if I wanted to chat to a child and parent and to put myself in a position to open up a conversation.*
>
> (Senior Nurse)

Working in a team where members have different levels of skill and expertise, nurses at the point of service delivery have to manage unpredictable patient needs with the complex temporal structures of the hospital. Owing to the turbulence on the wards, nurses' work rhythms were typically brisk and their contact with patients, often fleeting. Nurses recognized that this often made it difficult for patients to talk to them. Undertaking mundane work in quieter periods was a way of making themselves available to the patients. As Ersser (1997) has shown, patients value nurses making time for them.

DA: *I've seen you go round with your trolley – tidying up at the beginning of a shift.*

JUNIOR SISTER: *But I use that as a way of finding out if there's a problem [...] I won't spend long with everybody because some don't need you. It's just a case of 'Hello how are you getting on? How many times have you passed your water?' [...] I will also like tidy things up as I go [...] I think if it was me, at least if somebody's coming round all the time if there's something that they want to ask they are going to eventually ask somebody. So you just make yourself available.*

Strategic multi-tasking was also used by senior staff who performed mundane work – for example bed making – in order to unobtrusively supervise the work of juniors. As I described in Chapter 3, I employed a similar strategy in order to observe the ebb and flow of ward life for the purposes of the research.

To summarize, then, the turbulence of the ward environment does not lend itself to a rationalized division of labour. Given the interactive effects of time and space on nurses' work rhythms it would have been utterly impractical for nurses to divest themselves of all 'mundane work' activities and, as I hope my discussion of multi-tasking has shown, any attempt to do so ignores the subtleties and complexities of hospital nursing.

Hands-on care

While there seems to be a measure of agreement over the unskilled nature of certain activities routinely undertaken by nurses, the tensions between professional and management discourses reach their apogee around the question of the degree of skill involved in hands-on care. The holistic model of nursing advocated by the proponents of Project 2000 was clearly at odds with the aims of health service managers, who are concerned to cut labour costs and faced with a government imperative to reduce junior doctors' hours.

As I will describe in Chapter 6, irrespective of the jurisdictional claims made by the nursing leadership in the public arena, their ward-based colleagues spent as much time on paperwork as they did on patient work. Nevertheless, most valued hands-on nursing care highly and expressed regret that because of their other work pressures they were unable to spend as much time with patients as they would have liked. Davies (1995) calls this the 'polo mint problem', her choice of metaphor reflecting the fact that because nurses expend so much energy doing work around the patient, the practitioner role is not there. According to Davies, because nursing has always had to be accomplished with a variable and transient labour force, qualified nurses have found themselves supervising and managing the work of others who do most of the care delivery. Although Project 2000 went some way to stabilizing ward staffs there was little evidence of government commitment to the practitioner role – despite the rhetoric around the 'named nurse' initiative. The compromises that were made when Project 2000 was implemented led many to fear that nursing would be chiefly concerned with administration and management and thus fail to develop its clinical role. In their study of the implementation of Project 2000 in a single health authority, however, Elkan *et al.* (1994) found that in practice, because the HCA role was limited, qualified staff were able to retain an involvement in hands-on care but this often had to be combined with other management functions that greatly increased their burdens of work.

This picture described by Elkan *et al.* (1994) has obvious resonances with the situation of ward nurses at Woodlands. As we saw in Chapter 4, although nurses stressed the value of hands-on work it was also clear from their accounts that direct patient care activities involved emotional (Hochschild 1983; James 1989; Smith 1992) and physical labour that was difficult to sustain. Nurses who disliked patient contact work were considered deviant and derided for being lazy as this led to intolerable burdens for their colleagues. How do we reconcile these apparently paradoxical findings?

I suggest that although most of the nurses in this study were involved in clinical care, the pressures of work meant that they had few opportunities for sustained patient contact and hence the kind of relationship building felt to be a central reward of the job. Ersser (1997) has pointed to the ways in which shortages of staff made it difficult for nurses to make time for patients. It seemed to me that it was this aspect of their work nurses felt was missing rather than the clinical role *per se*.

> *I often say to my husband 'I wish I'd not done my training. I wish I was a health care assistant.' He says 'Well what do you mean?' and I say 'Well – it's a lovely job. You know they get in the bathroom.' I know they end up doing a lot of baths but that wouldn't bother me what-so-ever. I might have a different perspective if I was doing it all the time but you know to sit and have chance to talk to people and do their hair – it would be absolutely lovely.*

> (Staff Nurse – my emphasis)

Although reference to the rationing of medical treatment is now relatively commonplace in discussions of health care funding, it is highly unusual for 'care' to be referred to in these terms. Discussions of nursing tend to be framed instead in the language of 'standards'. This failure to include care in the rationing debates reflects the wider gendering of health policy and the invisibility of care in this masculine world. Care, unlike treatments, cannot be rationed because it cannot be seen. The corollary of this, moreover, is to deflect attention away from the rationing decisions nurses have to make on a daily basis and to focus instead on the implied inadequacies of nursing and nurses. The recent criticisms of Project 2000 are a case in point.

At Woodlands nurses' participation in direct patient care was highly variable, fluctuating according to the skill and grade mix of the staff on the ward and the peaks and troughs of the daily and weekly work rhythms. On weekdays, between 9 and 5, the demands on nursing staff were manifold. Most of nurses' effort went into co-ordination work, patient processing, liaising with doctors and communicating with patients' families and relatives. Nurses took the opportunity to undertake more hands-on care work at the weekend and on public holidays when the wards were typically quieter. The following observations were made on a Monday morning.

> Jane was in bay one doing the BMs [blood sugar monitoring]. The patients were remarking that they'd not seen very much of her today. Jane said, 'I was in here a lot yesterday because I wasn't busy. When I'm busy you don't see anything of me.'

During the week nurses had to ration their involvement in hands-on care. On both wards on the morning shift nurses and support staff initially worked towards the common purpose of getting patients up, helping them to wash and giving them their breakfast. After about 9 o'clock the division of labour became more differentiated. Support staff continued with hands-on care tasks and answered patients' call-bells. On Treetops ward qualified staff were preoccupied with preparing patients for theatre and processing new admissions to the ward. On Fernlea it was primarily the co-ordination of care activities such as liaising with doctors and making discharge arrangements that took nurses away from the hands-on care activities.

STAFF NURSE: Until about 9:30 you're with your patients doing the baths. That's when you get your patient contact. But then you have to leave the auxiliaries to finish off the baths because you have all the obs to do and the diary to sort out.

You spend all your time sorting out the diary. Then if you get an admission or, like this lady this morning who went really poorly, then that throws everything.

At night, when the working environment was typically less turbulent, nurses' involvement in direct care was again shaped by the other pressures on their time. At the beginning of the shift nurses were normally preoccupied with drug administration and patient observations. It was support staff, therefore, who settled patients and made them comfortable for the night. Once patient observations and drug administration were completed, however, direct patient care was shared between nursing and support staff.

The ward work rhythms affected the nursing-support staff interface in other ways. The need to adhere to organizational timetables, coupled with the uncertainty of the ward environment and the ever-present threat of an emergency, meant that nurses tried to keep themselves available in case their skills were needed. This had important implications for the division of labour between nurses and support staff. First thing in the morning nurses worked in the patient bay areas from where they were able to flexibly deploy their skills rather than 'getting tied up in the bathrooms'. It was support workers, therefore, who assisted patients in the bath. On the night shift – when there were typically only two qualified staff on duty – it was rare for nurses to be involved in the performance of last offices for similar reasons. This was a lengthy procedure that involved prolonged absence from the main ward area. As such this can be seen as denying nurses the opportunity to perform an important nursing ritual (Wolf 1988).[1]

Within this overall framework nurses appeared to employ a number of decision rules in selecting which patients for whom they were going to provide hands-on care. Priority was given to acutely ill patients. For example, on Treetops, the senior sister insisted that the nurses focused on those patients who had recently undergone major surgery. Allocating work in this way reflected the skill needed to manage a patient with a surgical wound, drips and drains. Nurses also concentrated on those patients where the provision of hands-on care allowed them to simultaneously engage in other skilled nursing activities. This is another example of nurses' strategic multi-tasking. In the following extract the staff nurse has decided to bath a patient in order to assess the condition of her skin.

STAFF NURSE: Have we got anyone else in our team?
HCA: There's Mrs Lawler.
STAFF NURSE: She's a blue. There's Mrs Wright. I said I'd do
    her because she says her bottom's sore.
HCA: And then that's us done.'

If the workload permitted, nurses also allocated themselves work for inter-personal reasons. Staff developed particular attachments to some patients.

> *Sometimes you find special patients who've been in a long time, the qualified prefer to do it [perform last offices], so it's the last thing that they can do.*
>
> (Auxiliary)

Thus far my analysis has focused on qualified nurses' involvement in caring processes on the ward and the factors that shaped the content of their work. The second thread in the debates about nursing work centres on the parameters of the support worker role.

What should the support worker be doing?

Many of the ward nurses had reservations about the HCA role and bemoaned their own lack of patient contact. Nevertheless, their concerns focused on the implications of dilution for their own work and the deni-gration of nurse training this implied, few actually questioned the skills of the support staff with whom they worked. Indeed, work was organized in ways that encouraged the routine blurring of the nurse–support worker boundary. In order to understand how the boundaries of the support worker role were accomplished at Woodlands we need to explore the interactive effects of two features of the work setting: the experiential biographies of staff and the temporal–spatial ordering of work.

Experiential biographies

The most striking feature about the allocation of work on both wards at Woodlands was its embeddedness in social relationships. The division of labour was based on trust and personal knowledge of staff skills, rather than formal occupational credentials.

> *I would decide individually not as a job, not as a 'Well she's a D grade staff or she's a health care assistant', I would take it as who they are and what experience they've got behind them.*
>
> (Junior Sister)

The 'experience' referred to in the above extract was of two kinds: expe-rience of work at Woodlands and personal life experience.

As I have observed, in the past, nursing shortages had resulted in an expansion of the role of auxiliaries. Several of the support staff had worked in the hospital for many years and, for the most part, their skills were acknowledged by those with whom they worked. Indeed some qualified members of staff even went so far as to express a preference for working with an experienced auxiliary with whom they had an established relationship rather than with an inexperienced registered nurse.

> *I had two good auxiliaries and I would trust them with things that I wouldn't trust my junior qualified nurses to do [...] I've had those two auxiliaries on with me and a junior staff nurse who's just qualified – and I think 'Who do I take to break with me and who do I leave on the ward?'*
>
> (Nurse Manager)

The informal skills hierarchy at Woodlands was also founded on personal life experience and again this could result in a division of labour that was at odds with the formal organizational plan. Here work was allocated on the basis of the assumed skills support staff brought into the workplace derived from their gender roles in the domestic division of labour. This was reflected in one ward sister's preference for 'mature' auxiliaries.

> Sister said that Paula was mature and this was another reason she thought she would be a good auxiliary.

In the following example a young staff nurse is talking about the involvement of an HCA in comforting bereaved relatives.

> [L]ike dealing with bereaved relatives, some people might think that she [HCA] shouldn't get involved, that it should be the staff nurses, but I think that she's had a lot more life experience than me and you know she perhaps could talk to them more. So I think get involved.
>
> (Staff Nurse)

This brings to mind the findings of James (1992b), who argues that in the hospice she studied there was almost an inverse law of status and skill in emotional labour: the young staff nurses relied on the four older auxiliaries who were described as the 'backbone' of the unit.

The temporal-spatial organization of ward work

On both wards much of the work was organized according to routines in which the work of nursing and support staff was clearly differentiated in time and space. For example, on Treetops when nurses performed patient observations, the support staff emptied catheters.

> *[W]hile I'm doing the catheters the qualified staff or students are doing the obs.*
>
> (HCA)

At night when the nurses administered medications and performed observations, support staff made and distributed milky drinks, and settled patients. Even when nurses and support staff worked together towards the common purpose of getting patients washed and ready for breakfast they mostly tended to different patients. Much of this work remained invisible, moreover, as it took place 'behind the screens' (Lawler 1991). On a number of occasions I observed that work routinely performed by the auxiliaries and HCAs was overlooked when they were not on duty. The extent to which the nursing and support roles were differentiated is highlighted by the observation that support staff who were new to the ward were sent to work with an experienced auxiliary or HCA and not a staff nurse.

> They have had a new nursing auxiliary start on the ward. It is her second shift [...] the senior sister was telling the auxiliary about things to remember – giving the men a shave, pulling the curtains back, collecting any empty medicine pots, making sure the medicine pots were dried properly.

SENIOR SISTER: Paula's [HCA] on tonight you can ask her. Do you know Paula?
AUXILIARY: Yes I worked with Paula yesterday.

Contemporary nursing ideology is highly critical of the routinization of ward work and a great deal of effort has gone into explaining the stubborn persistence of nursing routines. We saw in Chapter 4 that Menzies (1963) has suggested that the routinization of nursing work can be understood as a tacit strategy developed at the level of the organization in order to afford staff emotional protection from the demands of the work. More recently, other commentators have argued that routinization and task-allocation developed in order that permanent staff could control and cope with a transient student work force (Melia 1987; Proctor 1989; Davies 1995). By breaking patient care into a series of different tasks that are performed according to a pre-set routine, the sister creates a series of predetermined roles into which students could be slotted according to their stage of training.

Yet, although the problem of coping with a transient work force helps us to understand why the routinization of work was combined with hierarchical task allocation, it does not offer an adequate explanation of routinization itself. Indeed the *Mix and Match* review (DHSS 1986) found no clear relation in long-stay wards between a high proportion of qualified nurses and the practice of individualized patient care. My research suggests that nursing routines may be more fruitfully understood as a means through which nurses manage the multiple demands of the ward environment. It is a rational strategy for the efficient accomplishment of work, ensuring that all patients receive a minimally acceptable standard of care. Moreover, as Zerubavel (1979) has pointed out, the temporal structuring of hospital life constitutes a cognitive order providing staff and patients (Roth 1963; Fairhurst 1977; Zerubavel 1979) with a sort of 'repertoire' of what is expected, likely or unlikely to occur within certain temporal boundaries. The total absence of predictability would be psychologically intolerable (Moore 1963). Here, then, we can see that routines are both facilitating and constraining. They are necessary in order to manage the work but once established constrain the context in which the work is accomplished.

The routines on both wards afforded support workers considerable latitude over the performance of patient care, which, as we have seen, was central to nurses 'knowing the patient'. Support workers had to make daily decisions about what details ought to be brought to the nurses' attention.

[Y]ou have to work on your own initiative.

(Auxiliary)

HCA: [Y]ou get a lot of pressure – because you're the ones that are actually with the patients, so they come to you all the time and asking you if the patient's all right – 'Have you seen any breakages?', you know, 'Are they drinking?' and you've got to have all this for thirty-four patients – it's hard.

(HCA training day – Tape)

You like find out more about the patients – you know in my team – if anybody's got problems they usually can tell you and that, then it's to your discretion whether you pass it on.

(Auxiliary)

The division of labour on both wards cast support staff in a powerful role from where they were able to exercise a lot of indirect influence over both medical and nursing decisions. This brings to mind the classic treatment of Simmel (1950) of the complexities of superordination and subordination, and the interaction and exchange of influence that appearances conceal. Rather than a one-sided process of domination, hierarchy involves that 'in innumerable cases, the master is the slave of his slaves' (Simmel 1950: 185). The sociological literature confirms that support staff often control many aspects of the everyday running of wards, and through their judgements and reports, may have considerable influence on ward transfers, discharges, and the modification of diagnoses (Mechanic 1961; Scheff 1961; Strauss *et al.* 1964; Towell 1975; Wolf 1988). As we shall see in Chapter 7, similar observations have been made about the power of nursing staff vis-à-vis doctors.

These patterns of work were clearly at odds with the recommendations of the UKCC (1992) and formal organizational policy, which stated that support workers must work at all times under the direction and supervision of registered nurses. Nevertheless, where relationships were established, these arrangements had a number of advantages. For example, work could be accomplished more efficiently.

> I don't agree that a qualified member of staff should be bed-bathing a patient when there's ten admissions to be done because the HCA can't do that.
>
> (Junior Sister)

Given that considerable effort was absorbed by the need to manage the competing demands of the ward setting, nurses appreciated working with support staff who could be trusted to carry out work without supervision.

STAFF NURSE: It shouldn't be too bad this evening because, as I say the auxiliaries are good, they just get on.

STAFF NURSE: Say if I'm on with Jean I know I don't have to worry about things. But Dolly – although she's good she is still learning and so if I see if I'm on with her I know I shall have to work with her and keep an eye on what she is doing.

Support staff also valued the autonomy these working arrangements afforded them. On Treetops the efforts of certain of the senior nurses to exert more control over support staff resulted in tension.

> *[W]hat annoys me is – I know what I'm doing now – I know my role when I come on but you get one or two that like to sit in the*

chair and say 'You haven't done the catheters' and it's only half past nine and you don't do them until ten and it really annoys me because I've got other jobs until then and I know I'm going to do them but they're half an hour in front of you just so they can get that authority to actually say it.

(HCA)

While the permanent nursing staff appeared to accept the existing division of labour with support workers, students were rather more critical but their transient status and desire to 'fit in' (Melia 1987) with the ward team made them reluctant to express such criticisms openly. It could be argued that, because they typically worked more closely with support staff and also had an awareness of recent developments in nursing knowledge, students were well placed to judge support worker practice. We should, however, exercise a degree of caution in interpreting students' accounts. For, as Melia (1987) has shown, support staff pose particular problems for students' management of their occupational identity because of the extent to which their work overlaps.

Discussion

In this chapter I have examined the ways in which the boundary between nurses and support staff was being socially produced in two key domains at Woodlands. As we have seen, in certain arenas considerable negotiative effort was expended in order to demarcate the nursing and support worker roles and this yielded data amenable to the analysis of text and talk. The situation on the ward was quite different: here emphasis was given to the ward team rather than occupational difference and the practical concerns of the work setting resulted in a mode of work organization, which led to considerable blurring of the nurse–support interface. This division of labour was a largely tacit accomplishment, moreover, with surprisingly little face-to-face interaction between staff. As Strauss (1978) has acknowledged, when areas of social life are ordered by routines negotiation processes are minimized. Moreover, in long-standing relationships, understandings can be so well-established that negotiation is unnecessary.

To highlight the tacit aspects of nurses' and support workers' practices is not to claim that jurisdiction was wholly non-negotiated or that the support worker boundary was without limits. Although support workers had considerable latitude over hands-on tending on both wards, nurses maintained clear jurisdiction over the technical aspects of patient care. Support workers only undertook technical tasks when instructed to do so by staff nurses. It is somewhat paradoxical that despite the clear value accorded to basic nursing care activities by nurses they continued to exert the tightest jurisdictional control over the technical-medical dimensions of their work.

It is, however, difficult to assess to what extent the demarcatory practices of ward managers were oriented to by staff as autonomous constraints on their actions. In talking about the boundaries of their work, staff certainly shared many of the discursive resources employed by nurse managers. For example, reference was made to support staff having inadequate knowledge to carry out certain activities and emphasis was given to staff nurses' accountability for support worker practice. As I have shown, however, grass roots personnel also utilized alternative 'vocabularies of motive' (Mills 1940) that were not shared by managers and that were more frequently marshalled in their accounts as justifications for their actions. As we have seen, they often appealed to personal skills and experience and the best use of resources.

Miller (1997) has observed, that, one way of conceptualizing organizations is as a configuration of inter-related interpretative domains comprised of the 'local knowledge' (Garfinkel 1967; Geertz 1983; Gubrium 1989; all cited by Miller 1997) that setting members employ in making sense of their experiences. These 'normative frameworks' (Gubrium 1988) furnish discursive resources through which social reality is routinely interpreted and produced. Although they were members of the same organization and profession, nurse managers and ward level staff were clearly located, for the most part, in separate interpretative domains or social worlds (Strauss 1982). They had different interests, priorities and concerns, access to different discourses and operated within different constraints. This led them to formulate jurisdiction in distinctive ways: nurse managers were concerned with the social production of formal organization, whereas ward staff were preoccupied with the practical accomplishment of caring for the sick. The nature of the relations between ward level staff and nurse managers is considered in the next chapter.

6

THE NURSE–MANAGEMENT BOUNDARY

In the deliberations throughout the 1980s about the problem of health service governance, it was medicine's relationship with the state that was the primary target of policy makers' attentions. Nursing was largely ignored. At best, it was assumed that the model of management being proposed would have similar implications for nursing as it did medicine (Davies 1995). Yet the practice has been very different: new managerialism has had a far more profound effect on the work of nurses than it has that of doctors.

Although the discourse of professionalism is deeply rooted in its history, for a large part of its early occupational development, nursing, like the other non-medical 'professions', adopted a predominantly management route to occupational control. Beginning with the figure of the hospital matron, hierarchy had assumed a central place in the organization and regulation of nursing work. Since 1974 moreover, nursing had enjoyed a management structure that extended to all levels of the NHS. The Griffiths Report (DHSS 1983) changed all this. While hospital managers went to extraordinary lengths to encourage doctors into the management frame, nurses were effectively shut out. They lost the right to be managed exclusively by members of their own profession and fared very badly in the initial round of post-*Griffiths* appointments to general management posts (Harrison and Pollitt 1994). Nevertheless, as Harrison and Pollitt (1994) observe, nurse managers were quick to capitalize on *Griffiths'* emphasis on the patient and this brought a reorientation of nurse management towards issues of quality assurance. Many senior nurses have been appointed to posts concerned with such work (Strong and Robinson 1990; Harrison and Pollitt 1994).[1]

The patient-centredness of *Griffiths* and successive policy reforms may have created a welcome occupational niche for nurse managers, but the new consumer rhetoric has had its most penetrating impact on the work of staff at the point of service delivery. Many of the new managerialism's quality initiatives have centred on the service aspects of health provision and ward-based nurses have felt their effects acutely. It is nurses, for example, who have found themselves in the first line of defence in the rising tide of patient complaints. Furthermore, the creation of the purchaser–provider split and the introduction of the internal market generated a demand for information on many different aspects of service costs and quality; nurses have increasingly been expected to act as data collectors in the course of their everyday practice in order to support different aspects of quality audit. A rather less benign development in this period was the widespread introduction of systems imported from the US that claimed to 'measure' nursing care. Although the development of distinctive mono-professional scientific methods of audit were seen by many as an important marker of nursing's professional status, they also increased the potential for management control over nurses' work.

This chapter focuses on the nursing–management interface at Woodlands. In the first section I examine ward nurses' formulations of 'management' and the effects of the new managerialism on their daily practice. In the second part of the chapter I introduce the nurse managers responsible for implementing the initiatives considered problematic by ward staff, and explore the niche they occupied within the organization's overall management structure. I argue that these data suggest that the relationship between nurses and managers and the discourses of professionalism and managerialism is infinitely more complex than has hitherto been acknowledged.

The view from the wards

'Management' and 'the higher ups'

My attention was drawn to the significance of the nursing–management interface by nurses' complaints about the paperwork. This was by far the most common grievance staff expressed. From the perspective of ward personnel, paperwork was dirty-work (Hughes 1984). At one level, nurses' 'dirty-work designations' (Emerson and Pollner 1976) reflected their concerns about the increasing amount of paperwork and the demands it made on their time. At another level, nurses' complaints also indicated the paperwork's significance as a local symbol of the growing influence of the new managerialism over their everyday work.

Although it was nurses in management who were responsible for the implementation of the initiatives considered by grass-roots staff to be illegitimate, they were rarely singled out for explicit criticism. Rather, ward nurses referred to 'management', 'the hierarchy' and 'the higher ups' in a way that failed to differentiate nursing from general managers. In their formulations of the organization, 'management' were portrayed by ward staff as remote and anonymous, out of touch with the reality of ward life.

I think managers sit up there don't they and they don't really know what's happening on the ward and it makes me laugh really. They kinda troop on at Christmas and you think 'Who is this person?' You go 'Excuse me who are you?'. 'Well I'm the manager of the hospital.' 'Oh right I'm sorry I've no idea who you are.' And they troop on at Christmas and the patients don't know who they are they're not bothered about seeing them are they really. Yet they've no idea how a ward runs and what the staff are actually doing.

(Junior Sister)

You don't know who all these people are – the chaps who walk around in suits with name badges on. I don't know who half of them are. [...] They put people in to do the audit but not people to do the care! They might audit and say you've not got enough staff but they never give you any more.

(Senior Sister)

Sister Black recounted a story in which she had attended an open meeting held by the 'accounts man' – whose name nobody could remember. Sister Durham had also been at the meeting. Sister Black said that a charge nurse had raised the point that he was always over-spent on his budget because every year the nursing salaries went up by an increment. He explained that he tried everything he could think of to balance the books but he still ended up with the over-spend. The 'accounts man's' alleged response was stony and emotionless – 'I'm sure you'll find a way round it some way.' Sister Black said, 'He just cut him dead. He was completely emotionless. No "There's this or there's that or what about this?", just a "I'm sure you'll find a way round it some way." Everyone was flabbergasted.'

There are clear resonances here with the critical 'gender talk' described by Davies (1995), 'unknown a decade ago, which makes disparaging references to the new army of "men in suits", and questions the relevance of "grey suit" mentality to the NHS which generates and brings to bear an economic calculus that is devoid of human warmth and sympathy and that distances itself from the personal dilemmas and the suffering that those in the front-line of health care must face on a daily basis' (Davies 1995: 170). Managers were portrayed as wielding considerable and often arbitrary power over hospital staff, and, on a number of occasions throughout the period of the study this culture of suspicion was evident in the questions field actors raised about the research.

Staff Nurse said that in her view hospital management 'remember everything and turn it against you if they want to.'

Bev [staff nurse] introduced me to Sister Langworth. She asked me about the research. It's clear that when I mention the division of labour or occupational roles many people in the organization automatically think of skill-mix and less staff. Sister Langworth clearly assumed this. She was concerned as to how the information might be used by management to reduce the numbers even more. I tried to reassure her that that wasn't what I was about. She said 'Oh good so I haven't got to worry about giving a patient a bed pan then.'

Later on into the night Virginia asked me if management knew I would be spending the night on the ward. I said that I'd given them a timetable of my schedule of observations but I wasn't sure if the night sisters had seen it or not. Virginia said she was just wondering whether that was why they had four staff this evening when they usually had to work with three which is all they were funded for.

Paperwork and management control:
the paper construction of nursing.

[A]ny change to any procedure they bring a new piece of paper in that's twice as long. [...] It's ridiculous there's far too much paperwork and patients know because they'll say 'I've not seen you all afternoon'. [...] But it's when patients get to notice that you're doing a lot of paperwork they must know in their own minds that they're not given as much care, or time for the care. There's too much paperwork. I'd like to drop a big match on it all. To see it all go up.

(Staff Nurse)

Nurses' complaints about the volume of paperwork seemed well-founded: their work seemed to involve paper as much as it did patients. There was paperwork associated with the recording of essential clinical

102

information; paperwork involved in the ordering of clinical investigations and the making of specialist referrals; paperwork related to patients' discharge from hospital; paperwork that supported systems of audit; paperwork concerned with bed management and the movement of patients throughout the organization; and paperwork relating to the nursing record. Nurses had also developed their own informal recording systems in order to co-ordinate ward activity. Although nurses often couched their complaints in general terms, it was the paperwork they associated with the increased influence of the new managerialism that was held to be illegitimate. For example, many of the nurses were very critical of the documentation associated with the new patient discharge arrangements, which was part of a recently introduced quality initiative. This entailed a triplicate discharge letter and a quality assurance discharge check list that nurses had to sign to indicate that all the necessary arrangements had been made. Previously these details had simply been entered into the nursing kardex.

> *Like discharge letters. You don't have one any more there's two. One for the patient to take home, one for us to keep to say we've given them this letter to take home!*
>
> (Staff Nurse)

Another source of complaint was the additional paperwork that had been generated by the 'named nurse' initiative. All *Patient's Charter* standards were audited at Woodlands and the 'named nurse' constituted an important element in the quality standards agreed by the Trust's purchasers. As I outlined in Chapter 1, at one level, this government initiative had much in common with the professional vision of nursing, in which a designated practitioner assumes responsibility for the care of a given patient during his or her in-patient admission. Yet in the absence of sufficient resources to permit the implementation of a primary nursing model of care delivery, meeting the 'named nurse' quality standards on the ward meant that, for ward staff, the initiative was primarily a 'paper exercise'. As the following extracts indicate, being a 'named nurse' for a given patient had little influence on the ways nurses organized care.

STAFF NURSE: I think it's ['named nurse' initiative] a token gesture. OK if you admit a patient then you can ask them if they need a social worker or whatever and you can deal with it straightaway. But if something comes up during the patient's stay then somebody else might pick up on it and deal with it and refer them. Then if you happen to be on days off when the consultant decides to send them home then it's normally the nurse who did the ward round who sorts out the discharge. So it's a token gesture.

DA: *What about 'named nursing'. How does that work?*
STUDENT: [pulls a face] *I don't think it really does, does it? It's just a name on a piece of paper and at the end of the day I don't think patients are particularly bothered who sees to them or who sorts their problems out as long as they get sorted.*

The 'named nurse' – that again that's another paper exercise. It's a bit of a lottery the 'named nurse'. You may get a 'named nurse' and you may see her once and never again. It just seems to be a paper exercise.

(Nurse Practitioner)

Ward nurses' inability to implement 'named nursing' in a way that was in line with the professional ideal did not seem to cause them too much concern. As I described in Chapter 4, they employed a pragmatic system of work organization that embraced elements of both professional and management models. Additionally, many claimed that the majority of their patients had no interest in the 'named nurse' initiative or being involved in the planning of their care. Nevertheless, for audit purposes ward staff were obliged to demonstrate that they were satisfying this important *Patient's Charter* standard and this consumed their time and energy. For example, on Fernlea, the 'named nurse' for each patient was recorded in several places: on a white board in the main corridor, on the patient's identity bracelet, in the nursing kardex and on the patient's bed. In some areas, elsewhere in the Trust, nurses had developed business cards that they gave to their patients. All patients were to have met their 'named nurse' within 24 hours of admission to hospital but, owing to the demands of the work setting, this was frequently overlooked. When lulls in the work permitted, nurses could be observed going round all the patients in turn checking whether they had been allocated a 'named nurse'.

STAFF NURSE 1: You know when you do the kardexes later can you just check that everybody's got a 'named nurse'.
STAFF NURSE 2: OK. I think Jenny went through them the other day.

Although the nurses' actions were, to a considerable extent, an example of what Heimer (1998) has called 'ceremonial compliance', that is, they adopted a appearance of meeting the standard without honouring its spirit, these were nonetheless additional burdens of work on the nurses' time and a source of immense irritation.[2] In this sense then, the 'named nurse' initiative is a good example of how an apparent congruence between the discourses of professionalism and managerialism can spectacularly backfire in practice. Nurses felt bound by management initiatives to demonstrate the achievement of a professional model of practice in an environment that did not permit work to be organized in this way. Ironically, the extra work involved in doing 'ceremonial compliance' made the attainment of patient-centred care even less likely and created a work environment like that which Power (1999) describes as pertaining in the Soviet Union where detailed output targets created:

> a situation characterized by pathologies of 'creative compliance' (McBarnet and Whelan 1991), poor quality goods and the development of survival skills to show that, often impossible, targets were achieved.
>
> (Power 1999: 121)

Another area of tension at the nursing–management interface was the nursing record. Nurses' attitudes to the nursing record were equivocal. On both wards it appeared to be highly valued because of its relationship to contemporary professional ideologies and nurses were clearly loathe to criticize it directly. Yet despite the evident symbolic significance of the nursing process, nurses' increasing alienation from its utilization in practice was clear.

> *[T]hey're [care plans] a pain in the neck. I don't know. If I said that I didn't think care was any better for them. I don't know if I should say that really.*
>
> (Junior Sister)

In its current form, the origins of the nursing record lie in the nursing process. Although subject to some local variation, it comprises three main elements: a *pro forma* on which biographical information is recorded, a nursing history obtained, a nursing assessment undertaken, and discharge arrangements documented; a nursing care plan in which patients' problems or 'areas of concern' are identified and the appropriate nursing action to be taken is set out; and the nursing kardex, supposedly a contemporaneous record of the patient's progress.

The difficulties that have been encountered in integrating the nursing process into nursing practice are well-documented. While the nursing process has been successfully imposed on the syllabi for most areas of nurse education, with the exception of midwifery, the impact on practice has been universally disappointing (Dingwall *et al*. 1988). De la Cuesta (1983) has examined the implementation of the nursing process by ward staff in the US and UK. De la Cuesta argues that the major records in the nursing process experienced a different type of implementation. Nursing histories were instituted without great difficulty and consistently written, but they were regarded more as reference sheets containing patient information rather than as a foundation for nursing diagnosis and care planning.

According to De la Cuesta, the major barrier to the full implementation of the nursing process was the care plans, which were inconsistently written and had a medical/physical rather than a nursing focus. Nurses perceived care plans to be superfluous and argued that they had no time to write them. They also found it difficult to state the problems and express diagnostic concepts in writing. In her analysis, De la Cuesta moves beyond nurses' articulated reactions to the care plans and looks at organizational reasons for their scant success. She argues that although care plans are idealized by nursing theorists, in most hospitals they were destroyed after patients left and this devalued their importance. Moreover, for nursing staff the relationship of the care plan to the welfare of the patient was far from clear. Care plans were regarded as imposed formalities to be filled in when time was left to do them, something for administrative rather than practical purposes. De la Cuesta also points out that although it might not be explicitly stated, care plans imply accountability. Having committed a plan to paper, the nurse's deviations from it become all too apparent.

There have been major policy developments in the UK health care context since the time of De la Cuesta's study. More than ten years later ward-based nurses at Woodlands were still struggling to reconcile the ideals of the nursing process with their practice, but the reasons for this were rather different from those De la Cuesta describes. There were three principal grounds for nurses' estrangement from the nursing process at Woodlands: first, the increasing use of the nursing process as a management tool; second, the distortion of the content and purpose of nursing records by consumerism and litigation-consciousness; and third, the difficulty of employing the nursing process in a way which was useful in the working environment.

The nursing process was heralded as an important element in nursing's professional project. Yet while the detailed documentation of care made the nursing contribution more publicly visible it also opened the occupation to external scrutiny. As I pointed out in Chapter 1, part of the attraction of the nursing process from a management perspective is precisely the volume of paper it generates (Dingwall *et al*. 1988). At Woodlands, managers were using the nursing record as a quality indicator and this had the effect of indirectly controlling nursing work through standard setting. For example, nursing work was regularly audited using *Nurse Monitor*. Derived from a North American system, this is a tool concerned with the measurement of the 'quality' of nursing care and has been widely implemented throughout the NHS (Harrison and Pollitt 1994). It is a questionnaire-based instrument that has applicability to the nursing process; questions are answered by trained assessors (typically two per ward) and information is obtained from a number of different sources: the nurses, the patient, direct observation and, most importantly, the nursing record. Additionally, nurse managers in the study site had also developed their own local systems of audit in which the nursing record again figured prominently.

As Harrison and Pollitt (1994) point out, 'quality' is a highly politicized issue. It raises questions about how services are defined and measured and whose version is to prevail. At Woodlands there was a clear tension between the managers' efforts to enforce quality *standards* that had been agreed with the Trust's purchasers and the claims of nurses on the wards to provide *individualized* patient care. Nurses felt pressurized to routinely include certain problems on patient care plans in order to satisfy the quality assurance programme, irrespective of whether they had any relevance to the patient concerned.

STAFF NURSE: *[S]omebody went on a record-keeping day and they said we had to have 'bowels' on every one [care plan], we had to have 'psychological care' on every one [care plan] and something else on every single care plan.*
DA: *Health promotion!*
STAFF NURSE: [laughs] *Yes that's it. We did it because otherwise they say 'You haven't put that on' and you'd have to put it on.*

> *I think care plans are misused because management say that you need to then put on there's a problem – there's a certain problem – but each patient's an individual.*

(Junior Sister)

On Treetops, the satisfactory completion of the nursing record was rigorously enforced by the senior ward sister. Indeed standardized care plans existed for the main surgical cases seen on the ward, which nurses diligently transcribed at the weekend when the ward tended to be quieter. Initially staff on Fernlea had also succumbed to the pressures for standardization. At the time of the fieldwork, however, they were becoming increasingly prepared to defend their right to plan care individually.

> *[T]hey were telling us what to put on – when they don't know patients, they've not admitted them, they've not looked through their assessment. So how do they know whether they suffer from constipation or they need health education or whatever?*
>
> (Staff Nurse)

It is important to be clear that what is being referred to here is the implications of managerialism on nurses' record-keeping not their clinical work. The need to satisfy quality standards that were audited via the record, imposed on ward staff a particular accounting practice as a work obligation. The result was the paper construction of a management version of 'quality' nursing care (or at least ward nurses' perceptions of it), which was at odds with the patient-centred vision to which they subscribed.

The satisfactory completion of the nursing record was further reinforced by the new consumerist ethos in health care and the attendant fear of litigation. Even though there are many aspects of the caring process over which nurses have little control, the elaborate planning of care increases the personal accountability of the nurse for its delivery (De la Cuesta 1983; Bowers 1989; Salvage 1995). De la Cuesta observes that the implied accountability of care plans resulted in a reluctance on the part of nurses to commit their plans to paper. Nursing staff at Woodlands were acutely aware of the accountability implied by the care plans, however, and their satisfactory completion was ensured through standard setting. Every patient had to have a care plan within 24 hours of their admission. Nurses managed their implied accountability for care by utilizing the care plans in order to structure their written records. An entry was made for each 'problem' identified, and, as a consequence, kardex entries were lengthy.

> *You've got to answer every problem so that you've stated that you know about that problem. That's all you're trying to prove that you know about their bowels, that you know whether they've had a wash and you're trying to prove it in your little green sheet that you know. Whereas you don't know half of the time until you ask them!*
>
> (Staff Nurse)

[E]veryday people are going round and writing the same old thing you know. 'Patient has had a bath this morning', 'No complaints of pain' when they didn't have any complaints of pain yesterday. Do you know what I mean? It's like the same gumff every day. [...]. People are so frightened of missing something and so frightened of it coming back to them that we record the same old thing every day. And I think it's too much.

(Staff Nurse)

As a result of the combined effects of a management emphasis on quality assurance and a consumerist climate in which staff were ever-fearful of the threat of litigation and patient complaints, considerable nursing energy went into maintaining a 'satisfactory' nursing record. This supports the findings of Annandale (1996) who interprets the 'excessive' documentation undertaken by nursing staff as a defensive strategy in a climate of anxiety about risk management. Of course nurses may well have been able to justify the time they spent on paper-work if they believed that the nursing record helped them in their daily practice and had advantages for patient care. In reality, however, the pressures of work on the wards meant nurses were rarely able to consult the nursing record. The only time they referred to the care plans was when they came to write the kardexes. Thus although care plans might have served as a useful *aide memoire* to ensure aspects of care were not overlooked, nurses rarely consulted them before care was delivered.

The nursing record's lack of utility in the routine work of ward staff was not simply a reflection of the guise it had assumed under manageri-alism however. It also stems from the discontinuity in the professional vision of nursing on which the nursing process is premised and the workplace reality of hospital wards. As I have argued, the nursing process is based on a model of professionalism taken from private-prac-tice with built-in assumptions about a one-to-one relationship between professional and client. Nurses on hospital wards, however, have to simultaneously manage a number of individual cases and co-ordinate patient care with diverse, and often conflicting, organizational timeta-bles. Care plans were of little help to the busy nurses in managing their work priorities.

They do a record-keeping day here and they say that [...] You should go on and you should look at your care plans and you know exactly what care to give to that patient. But I'm sorry in an ideal world, realistically if as soon as you walk on that ward and you start walking round looking at care plans the buzzers are going, the breakfasts arrive, people want a wash, they want to get out. You can't do it. You'd get half way down and then what? Somebody might have a colonoscopy booked for 10 o'clock and by the time you've got there it's too late and they've missed their enema that they should have had at 8 o'clock because you started at the other end instead of that end.

(Staff Nurse)

Nurses had developed their own informal methods in order to manage the work. Both wards had a diary system and although the schemes varied in their finer details the most important feature was that, unlike the care plans that related to the needs of a single patient, the ward diaries referred to the totality of nursing work for the shift. In utilizing the diaries, nurses were able to see at a glance the activities to be carried out, and prioritize their work accordingly.

[Y]ou can see what needs doing straightaway and see what you can leave until later. I like that.

(Student)

Of course there are other possible reasons for nurses' failure to use the nursing process in their routine practice. The nursing process was initially developed as a teaching device, and it is questionable as to how useful the detailed recording of the problem solving approach is for an experienced nurse. It has been suggested that the stages of the nursing process – assessment, planning, intervention and evaluation – inadequately represent how nurses practise (Benner 1984; Lawler 1991). As Savage (1995) points out, much of nurses' knowledge is 'embodied' and many nursing actions are, arguably, an intuitive response to the moment (Meerabeau 1992). For the most part, qualified nurses at Woodlands maintained that they knew patients' needs without having to refer to the care plan. They relied on nursing hand-over for information about non-routine aspects of patients' care and expected work colleagues to keep them up-to-date with any important relevant developments. Handover took the form of a narrative and anecdotal story-telling, and contained information that could never have been captured in the nursing kardex. Parker *et al.* (1992) have also observed the divergence in the information contained in the nursing notes, compared with that which is transmitted at handover. In Parker *et al.*'s study patients' notes centred on the body, whereas at handover nurses discussed the affective and subjective elements of patient care. At Woodlands, nurses placed a great deal of importance on knowing patient details without having to consult the record. As we saw in Chapter 4, staff felt foolish if they were asked about a patient and were unable to provide the information. There are certain parallels here with Dingwall's (1977a) study of health visitor training in which not using the record was a mark of professional expertise. Unlike Dingwall's health visitors, however, nurses' non-use of the record was not a self-conscious attempt to demonstrate their skill. More often than not it was simply a case of there being insufficient time. Nevertheless, managing without the care plan was essential in order to function in the ward working environment and not 'knowing the patient' without having to consult the record was felt to reflect badly on one's competence, particularly in front of doctors or relatives.[3]

In this section I have explored ward nurses' formulations of hospital management and the impact of the new managerialism on their everyday work. I have highlighted the importance of paperwork as a local symbol of the managerialist ethos and increased control and scrutiny of nursing work. In the second part of this chapter I want to examine the social worlds (Strauss 1982) of nurse managers at Woodlands who had the task of implementing the initiatives ward staff found so objectionable.

The view from nurse management

The nurse managers

Excluding the Director of Nursing, who was a member of the Trust Executive Board, there were ten nurses in management posts at Woodlands. I was fortunate to have the opportunity to undertake interviews with eight of them. Although they came together for meetings and shared many common concerns, for analytic purposes they may be considered as two distinct groups: traditionalists and strategists.

Traditionalists

The four traditionalist nurse managers were all members of clinical management teams and were responsible for nursing management within their particular directorates. All were mature women who had reached their posts by virtue of their extensive nursing experience. None had formal management training and there was a feeling amongst this group, that this type of manager was an endangered species. At the start of the research each clinical management team was headed by a clinical director – who was a consultant – and assisted by the nurse manager and general manager as equals. In one directorate, the post of nurse and general manager were combined. During the course of the research, however, the hospital Chief Executive gave each directorate the opportunity to alter its management structure making the general manager the direct deputy to the clinical director, effectively relegating the nurse manager to a junior role. Not all of the clinical management teams elected to make this change and in some that did, it made little practical difference because of the personalities involved. Nevertheless, many saw the move as sounding the death knell for nurses in management at Woodlands.

Strategists

This group of nurse managers were primarily concerned with Trust-wide strategic and developmental issues. They can be considered as two distinct groups, divided by gender. The first group referred to themselves as 'the fledglings'; illustrating their belief that they were being groomed for higher posts by the Director of Nursing. All in their late twenties or early thirties, these four women had been ward sisters early in their careers and had undertaken, or were in the process of undertaking, diplomas or degrees in nursing. Each had responsibility for specific areas of nursing practice: Project 2000 and professional development, tissue viability, infection control and nursing audit. They formed a cohesive group and shared an office on the same corridor as the Director of Nursing. The adjacent office housed the two other strategic managers: the IT project leader who was responsible for the implementation of a computerized ward management system, and the Quality Manager. Both were male and in their late thirties.

Professionalism, managerialism and pragmatism: nurse managers' vision(s) of nursing

Nursing, as we have seen, has a long history of management hierarchy and nurse managers are often identified as a distinct segment within the nursing work force. Writing in the mid 1970s, for example, Carpenter (1977) identified 'new managers' as one of three main groups within nursing. According to Carpenter, the 'new managers' emerged after the Salmon Report (Ministry of Health 1966) and functioned according to an industrial model of management rather than a collegial model of professional behaviour. The second group Carpenter identified was the 'new professionals', these were clinical specialists who appropriated the more complex parts of nursing work. The third group – 'rank and file' – represented the mainstream of nursing. Ten years later, as the professional vision of nursing moved into the ascendant, Melia (1987) suggested the existence of a fourth group: the 'academic professionalizers'. This group are to be found, in the main, in academic circles and they tend to be removed from patients. According to Melia, a major cleavage within nursing is the division between service and education sectors. The education segment is concerned with the production of competent registered nurses, capable of independent practice and professional judgement, whereas the concerns of the service segment are more immediate: the accomplishment of nursing work.

> Nurses who become managers are managers first and foremost. Their definition of nursing problems and solutions arise out of organizational need rather than a preoccupation with nursing interventions and patients' rights to health.
>
> (Perry 1993: 71, quoted by Bergen 1999)

Strong and Robinson (1990) seem to provide some support for this characterization, observing that many of the new nurse managers they interviewed had a very different approach to the professional vision.

> ASST UGM/DNS: The CNA came round one of the wards because there'd been a lot of complaints from patients and pressure sores were going up – we've got a very low level of staffing. She said that in the future maybe we'd need fewer staff – but that they would be much better trained and more adaptable, 'Wouldn't that be best?' I said, 'Fine, but four nurses can't do the work of six.' It's the nature of the work. We need lots of pairs of hands when we're dealing with very dependent people.
>
> (Strong and Robinson 1990: 86)

> DEPUTY DGM/CNA: The nursing process has had an extremely disturbing effect. It's been under-rated in its complexity and over-rated in its productivity. Above all it's never been evaluated. Like most things in nursing, it's been put in *ad hoc*. There's never been any parallel system of evaluation.
>
> (Strong and Robinson 1990: 87)

For certain purposes it is useful to consider nursing in terms of its different constituent segments. As I suggested in Chapter 5, in a very real sense different members of the occupation inhabit diverse social worlds or 'interpretative domains' (Miller and Holstein 1993). They have different concerns and interests, operate within different kinds of constraint and employ different interpretative resources and vocabularies of motive. In this section we explore the social world of nurse

113

managers at Woodlands and discover a rather more nuanced reality than previous formulations of this segment of the occupation have indicated.

With the exception of the Quality Manager (who will be discussed later) one of the things that struck me very forcibly about the nurse managers was the prominence of the discourse of professionalism in the language they employed and in the vision of nursing they promoted. This was a surprise; I had expected to find, as had Strong and Robinson (1990), that nurse managers would embrace a service rather than a professional model of nursing. Contrary to my expectations, however, I found that in their conversations with me and in the course of their everyday work, nurse managers espoused many of the ideals of the 'new nursing'. For example, they emphasized the value of bedside nursing and underlined the importance of a holistic approach to care.

> *I still feel that perhaps the most skilled nurses are the ones who should be sometimes doing the bed baths and turning patients, making them comfortable because in all of that they're observing and noting things and building up a relationship aren't they – to then carry it further.*
>
> (Director of Nursing)

> *A bed bath gives you an opportunity to do so much more doesn't it. You gather so much information from doing a bed-bath. It's a long time since I've done one but you do – you're doing so much more than just washing the patient's skin aren't you? I think it's quite an art – doing a bed bath. [...] There is quite an art to washing someone in bed and keeping them comfortable while you're doing that.*
>
> (Strategist)

> *[I]t's all to do with the intuitive thinking about when you're doing tasks with patients like bathing them and bed-bathing them you're not just doing the job for the job's sake you're doing it because you're looking at all the things that make up that patient that inform your intuitive reasoning about what makes you recognize when patients' conditions are either improving or deteriorating.*
>
> (Strategist)

Nurse managers' discourses were, however, tempered with a fair degree of pragmatism. Although they were committed to many of the 'new nursing' ideas, they were realists and well aware of the constraints within which their colleagues on the shop-floor worked. They talked about the importance of nurses striving for their ideals but acknowledged that sometimes circumstances forced uncomfortable compromises. We have already seen, for example, that nurse managers recognized that the hospital had inadequate staffing numbers to support primary nursing and opted for a team nursing model instead.

> *But within team nursing the ideal would be primary nursing and we set off in the first instance, there were all these wonderful ideas in the nursing press about doing primary nursing and you'd go to Steve Wright's unit and he's promoting all this wonderful work and you think yes there's some good ideas there and you come back and you think I can't do primary nursing I've got two trained staff and I'm one of them!*
> (Strategist)

> *I don't know how purist you can be. You've got to be flexible and adaptable [...] I think what you've got to do is say 'OK if for today primary nursing or team nursing comes collapsing in around our ears then it does but what we have to do is to pick up the pieces afterwards and look at why it did and not just say, 'Oh gosh it's collapsed therefore it doesn't work.'*
> (Strategist)

Although the nurse managers employed a pragmatic as well as a professional discourse, they were also at pains to distance themselves from general and medical managers within the organization. They were, first and foremost, nurses.

> *I mean I'm basically a nurse although I might be in a managerial role. It's nursing for nursing – and I'm sorry that's my attitude to it and I object to seeing people coming in to erode my nursing role.*
> (Traditionalist)

> *Nursing as far as I am concerned has always been my reason for being in whatever post I've been in. Nursing's still important to me because the profession of nursing is important and professional standards[...] [W]hen we were becoming a Trust we were encouraged as very senior nurses not to appear 'nursey'. Now I was just too old to change and I found that quite difficult I expect because I feel somebody has to be nursey*

and put a professional point of view forward even if you take on other roles and responsibilities and do work that you wouldn't normally have done.

(Director of Nursing)

It was clear that the nurse managers saw themselves as different from non-nurse managers within the Trust. They frequently made disparaging references to the medical and general management 'camps' which they portrayed as possessing considerable power.

[I]t's a constant struggle. Nothing that is achieved by nurses is achieved without an awful lot of effort, whereas [...] if you're in either the medical camp or the general managers' camp resources are very readily available whereas nurses!

(Strategist)

Debbie [Strategist] talked about the importance of the hospital social life. She said that the marketing manager came for one job – 'played cricket with the Chief Executive and then landed the marketing manager's job.' She said there was a bit of an old boys' network in operation.

These hospital management boards and things like that – it's difficult to get nursing things on the agenda. You know, I should have been on the [?TEG] agenda this month and they've sort of like said 'There's too much on the agenda'. [...] So we'll see what happens next month. So you know I think it's CMTs that have the last say and clinical management teams are headed by the consultants and managers aren't nursing as such.

(Strategist)

Many of the nurse managers were explicitly critical of the new managerialism: protocols, the need for hard data, the *Patient's Charter*, and organizational impression management (Goffman 1959).

Everything has to have a report behind it these days. Every decision that is taken. It's as if we can never do anything without paper.

(Traditionalist)

Nothing's right unless you produce a statistic. [...] I know that them staffing levels [...] aren't adequate. My word's not good enough. I've got to prove it on a piece of paper. I find that quite ludicrous.

(Traditionalist)

It's ['named nursing'] a task and it's a chore and you some-times wonder if it's worthwhile. It's something that's been imposed on you by government that you've got to do. It's not something that you've taken on yourself and I think there's a difference when something's imposed on you from when it's something you're interested in doing yourself. They do try to do it but at the end of the day you get so many patients you just exhaust yourself. You know what are we achieving here? Why are we trying to achieve it when it's not achievable and then you think – what's the point?

(Strategist)

The one exception to this overall characterization of the ward managers' w*eltanschauung* was the Quality Manager. He employed a predomi-nantly managerialist discourse. Waiting in his office in order to inter-view him I noticed that his bookshelves contained a number of management texts, including *In Search of Excellence* (Peters and Waterman 1982)[4] and *Thriving on Chaos* (Peters 1987). This interview was quite unlike any other I carried out; he berated the health profes-sions for their tribalism and talked about the need to think innovatively about the health services, division of labour.

[I]f you've got a patient-focused environment, then you work round what is in the best interests of the patient not what's in the best interests of the professional groups. I think we should be working as a team. Not just perhaps trying to work as one professional or another and to score points over one another.

(Quality Manager)

I think we could be more efficient, and I think this is what hospitals in America have found, where they have someone going round siting all the IVs. You can be very efficient at getting it done.

(Quality Manager)

Professionals want to exert their power and that comes from their own egos or their own professional bodies. [...] So they have power too which is often in tension with that of the organization.

117

Then you look at the patient – the power they have – the patient has got power. The patient can say yes or no – 'No I don't want you to treat me. This is what I want you to do for me.'

(Quality Manager)

In contrast to the other nurse managers then, the Quality Manager appeared to embrace much of the new management ethos. Within the nurse manager group, however, he was an isolated case. Moreover, he had no direct responsibility for implementing the management initiatives derided by front-line staff, and unlike the other nurse managers, had little contact with clinicians.

Mediating the nursing–management boundary

Despite feeling deeply uncomfortable about many of the initiatives they had been asked to take forward within the organization, the nurse managers clearly felt relatively powerless to resist them.

Junior doctors' hours are going to reduce anyway whether we like it or not. It's something that Parliament is quite keen to do and it's going to happen [...] If your patient needs an Amino-phylline drip there and then I think it's inevitable and it's a must that we do it.

(Strategist)

One of the ways they appeared to have accommodated themselves to these constraints was by taking control of initiatives as they arose and trying to use them to further the vision of pragmatic professionalism to which they subscribed. So, for example, the need to implement the 'named nurse' initiative was used to give an added impetus to the implementation of team nursing in the study site; the junior doctors' hours initiative was used as an opportunity to underline the value of holistic care; and, as we saw in Chapter 5, the introduction of HCAs allowed nurse managers to shore-up occupational boundaries and underline nurses' responsibility and accountability.

Nurse managers played an important role in translating directives originating outside of nursing for the purpose of disseminating them to rank-and-file staff. In this sense, they were important mediators of the nursing–management interface, deftly traversing the tensions between professional and management discourses.[5] On the in-service training days I attended I noticed how nurse managers formulated external initiatives in ways that allowed both association and disassociation.

Greta pointed out that the government had said that this ['named nurse'] was the way in which they were going to have to nurse. She pointed out that the *Patient's Charter* didn't outline how nurses should go about it. [...] Greta said that in her view the only way truly to latch the 'named nurse' scheme onto care delivery was to tie it to primary nursing. However, the government cannot do that, she pointed out, because of the cost implications for care. The financial implications steered the government away from using the phrase 'primary nursing'.

('Named nurse' study day)

GRETA: But one of the things that we've been asked to do and we can't really get out of it is that we've got to monitor and report back to District about how well we're doing with this particular target. Not only because it's in *The Vision*[6] but more importantly it's in the *Patient's Charter* and everything that's in there we have to audit! So just independent people as far as I'm aware were walking round asking patients questions.

('Named nurse' study day - Tape)

Debbie tried to present where audit fitted in within the overall structure. She explained that 'the District were very hard driving about what they see as audit'. She said that the need was to try and 'influence that from the bottom up because if we don't we're going to have audit imposed on us.'

(*Vision for the Future* study day)

An interesting feature of these extracts is the way in which the nurse managers' formulations are oriented to a model of constraint. This is a useful device by which nurse managers are able to drive management initiatives forward while simultaneously constructing a degree of professional distance from them.

The case of audit

The implementation of audit in the study site is one example of how nurse managers attempted to modify elements of the new managerialism for professional purposes. At the time of the research, considerable effort was being expended developing a collegial model of audit to replace the old-style hierarchical one. A number of systems of audit which, in the past, had been undertaken by external agents or line managers, were now being carried out by peers at ward level. Moreover, rather than have nurse managers instigate practice developments in response to the audit, front-line staff were encouraged to develop their own 'action plans'.

Of particular interest here is the 'named nurse' audit. The original audit tool had been developed by the Quality Manager and was oriented to assessing the extent to which nurses were achieving the primary nursing ideals associated with the 'named nurse' initiative. It relied heavily on patients' answers to a series of questions relating, for example, to whether they knew the name of their 'named nurse' or whether they'd seen their care plan. When the audit indicated that nurses were not achieving the *Patient's Charter* standard (as measured by the tool in existence at the time) two of the strategist nurse managers were asked by the Director of Nursing to develop a series of training days to improve performance. As part of the process of taking the 'named nurse' initiative forward the nurse managers worked with the ward nurses who attended the training programmes to develop the original audit tool. Having acknowledged that implementation of the 'named nurse' in any meaningful sense was not possible given the staffing levels on the wards and that patients themselves had little interest in it, their aim was to develop a system that would at least give credit to the efforts of ward staff in achieving 'ceremonial compliance' with the standard.

STRATEGIST [DEBBIE]: Basically we tried to simplify the whole thing ['named nurse' audit] and also put it in the hands of the nursing staff because they were doing a lot of work towards the 'named nurse' but they weren't always getting rewarded for it.

('Named nurse' study day)

STRATEGIST [GRETA]: Observation of the environment – things like picture boards, name boards, bracelet identification on the patients, business cards. Anything that has the 'named nurse' advertised if you like would be given credit for. I think Sister Black last time produced a little A4 booklet, piece of paper – 'Welcome to Daffodil Ward. I am your 'named nurse'.' So that would have gone down as something extra. Because we felt that even though a patient might not be aware of it yet they've done everything that you could possibly do you should still get credit for that and not just relying on the patient's information.

('Named nurse' study day – Tape)

A further interesting theme on this and other days in the in-service training programme was the emphasis nurse managers placed on the importance of professional knowledge in the production of hard data. They clearly recognized, as have Gubrium and Buckholdt (1979), that:

> The definitional and interpretative work necessarily engaged in by data gatherers shows that whatever rigour and concreteness the data come to have once they have been collected is not simply a result of the technical soundness of the procedures involved. The work as such of data gatherers in generating hard data, literally constitutes – indeed produces – the rigour and concreteness the data is assumed to have.
>
> (Gubrium and Buckholdt 1979: 121)

In these sessions nurse managers routinely appealed to nurses' privileged knowledge of service realities in contrast to the decontextualized knowledge of general managers.

> Debbie recounted a story about *Nurse Monitor* in which the man who was doing the assessment had come to a ward [...] and while he was there a patient urinated on the floor – it was a care of the elderly ward. Because there was urine on the floor near the toilets the man had assessed the ward environment as unsatisfactory. Debbie expressed her frustration at this simplistic view – arguing that in wards of that type people did urinate on the floor and if nurses were wiping up urine the whole time then what else would they not be doing.
>
> (*Vision for the Future* study day)

Interestingly, in underlining the importance of a professional interpretative frame, the nurse managers were not appealing to an idealized model of professional practice, but a pragmatic one based on a grass-roots understanding of the work context.

At one level, then, the system of audit being taken forward by senior nurses in the study site was based on a collegial, rather than a management model, founded as it was on the contrast between insider professional knowledge and the inappropriate interpretative lens of 'outsiders'. At another level, however, the approach also entailed a rejection of many of the professional standards of care on which the traditional systems of nursing audit were based and the introduction of alternative quality indicators rooted in the work context. Nurse managers hoped that this new model of audit would produce hard data that did justice to the nursing contribution to health provision given the constraints within which they worked. Yet while these developments also brought nurses much closer to the medical system of audit amongst nominal peers than had previously been the case, the results of nursing audit were still made available to managers and the Trust's purchasers. Fully cognisant of the interpretative practices involved in doing audit, those nurses involved in the process felt this burden of responsibility acutely.

NURSE PRACTITIONER: It's awful doing this because you know for yourself that you don't like it being done – you don't like to question your colleagues' practice.

Clare Black (Sister) expressed concern that the whole exercise was highly subjective and that her opinion could differ widely from someone else doing it.

Reflecting over lunch on the experience of doing the *Nurse Monitor* audit the following conversation ensued:

SISTER BLACK: Where are all these quality managers? Shouldn't they be doing this? We're doing their job for them. We've got enough to do in our own areas. [...]

DA: But if it was the managers wouldn't that feel like big brother watching you?

SISTER BLACK: I think all this does is puts staffs' backs up against each other.

NURSE PRACTITIONER: We could all have good records in an ideal world with one patient but you don't, you just put down what you can, don't you?

SISTER BLACK: There are so many audits. Audit of this and audit of that. We're doing an audit of elective surgery beds at the moment. It's just something else to fill in.

Thus it would seem, that despite the nurse managers' efforts to introduce a professional model of audit, clinical staff perceived this to be divisive. Under the old system, if the audit was critical of nursing care then staff could at least blame the anonymous man in the grey suit who had little understanding of the workplace reality at ward level, but peer assessment that remained open to external scrutiny clearly felt like an entirely different matter, and was yet another job clinical staff were being expected to take on without additional resources.

Conclusions

In this chapter I have examined the nursing–management interface at Woodlands. Beginning with the social worlds of the wards, I explored the critical 'gender talk' that ward nurses employed in their formulations of management. I then went on to look at the effects of the new managerialism on the work of front-line staff. I pointed to the significance of paperwork as a local symbol of general management's growing influence over the everyday work of health care professionals. I have argued that, although the new managerialism did not directly control nurses' clinical practice, the need to satisfy certain quality initiatives had imposed on them particular methods of accounting for their work that were time consuming and a distraction from patient care. Yet nurses' complaints about the paperwork did not indicate a straightforward tension between the discourses of professionalism and managerialism, however. Indeed a number of the quality initiatives that were considered most problematic by staff at the front-line were those that resonated most strongly with the 'new nursing' ideals. Because the professional vision of nursing is grounded in a very different reality from the one in which hospital practitioners function, its enforcement by standard-setting resulted in a time-consuming process of ceremonial compliance, leaving staff even less time for clinical activity. Here then, the apparent convergence of management and professional discourses has had a profoundly negative effect on ward level nursing.

In the second half of the chapter I explored the social worlds of nurse managers. I argued that, with the exception of the Quality Manager, the nurse managers had embraced much of the professional vision of nursing. They were supportive of many of the 'new nursing' ideals, for example, and their sense of nurses as autonomous professionals was strong. At the same time, however, they were pragmatists; they knew the constraints within which nurses worked and recognized that compromises were inevitable. Although they had certain reservations about many of the initiatives with which they were charged, they felt unable to withstand them. Instead they adopted a strategy of mediation in which management initiatives were used for professional purposes. So for example, even though they accepted that the 'named nurse' initiative could not be implemented because of the staffing levels, they developed the 'named nurse' audit tool so that it reflected the efforts being expended at ward level to accomplish ceremonial compliance. We also saw how they were implementing a new – non-hierarchical – system of audit in which the interpretations of ward level staff were considered central. This entailed a rejection of many of the professional standards implicit in the old audit tools and the implementation of a more realistic assessment of the quality of nursing care, which took into account the limiting effects of the work environment.

Despite the nurse managers' efforts to implement a professional rather than a management model of regulation, ward nurses' sense of hierarchy was strong. On a number of occasions several of the strategist managers berated ward level staff for their inability to challenge the system. Others were more sympathetic, pointing out that nurses had experienced hierarchy for so long they could not be expected to act and think like autonomous professionals over-night. Arguably, however, the reticence of ward level staff was grounded in rather more concrete concerns. Levels of unemployment in the locality were high, and a large number of the nurses in the study were the main wage earners in their household. The overriding concern for most of them was to provide the best patient care they could within the constraints in which they worked without finding themselves in court or rocking the organizational boat in the process. Although at times they employed a professional discourse and were interested in professional issues the furtherance of nursing's professional project was not top of their daily list of 'to dos'.

The data examined here also illustrate the complexity of the relationship between the discourses of professionalism and managerialism and nursing and management. Past formulations of nurse managers have tended to characterize this segment of the occupation as preoccupied with service concerns. The views of nurse managers at Woodlands suggest that at one level this still holds true, but that professional considerations also figure prominently in their interpretative horizons. I have suggested that nurse managers at Woodlands worked with a pragmatic model of professionalism that took into account the realities of the work setting. The one exception to this was the Quality Manager who embraced a managerialist discourse that was clearly at odds with his nursing colleagues.

To what extent the differences I have described here are representative of nursing management elsewhere is difficult to judge. Traynor's (1999) recent examination of the discourses employed by nurse managers also indicates the need for a more sophisticated understanding of nurses in management. His data reveal that some nurse managers had unequivocally embraced the rhetoric of new public management, but there were others who expressed more hesitant views. One issue of particular interest is the extent to which this is a gendered division. I was unable to interview the IT manager – who was the only other male nurse manager in the organization – and, even if I had, one more interview would have done little to have increased my confidence in my findings. It does, however, suggest a very interesting area of further research.

7

THE NURSE–DOCTOR
BOUNDARY

In this chapter I examine the ways in which the boundary between nurses and doctors was being produced at Woodlands. As outlined in Chapter 1, developments in nursing and medical education and the health service reforms had created significant jurisdictional ambiguity for nursing and medical staff. On the one hand, management discourse emphasized the need for nurses to undertake doctor-devolved work in order to improve the hours and working conditions of junior doctors and contribute to the achievement of organizational efficiencies. On the other hand, nursing's professional discourse underlined the occupation's difference from medicine and, in attempting to reintegrate caring activities into the core professional nursing role, it was challenging the traditional status hierarchy that elevated 'technical' over caring work in the provision of health services. Both versions of nursing found their proponents within the occupation, and, adding yet another layer of complexity, those who supported the devolution of 'doctors'' work to nurses often employed the rhetoric of 'profession' in legitimating their position.

The changing medical–nursing boundary at Woodlands:
an overview

During the period of the study, efforts were being made to realign the formal division of labour between nurses and doctors at Woodlands. A number of nurse practitioner posts had been founded that involved nurses undertaking work that, in the past, had been the remit of doctors. These new positions had all been created in the context of the junior doctors' hours initiative and they covered a range of clinical areas such as urology, rheumatology, IV cannulation, pain control, colposcopy and general surgery. The *New Deal* had also provided the impetus for a more general realignment of medical and nursing work: ward-based nursing staff were being encouraged to develop their scope of practice to incorporate activities such as the administration of intravenous antibiotics, venepuncture, ECGs, male urethral catheterization and intravenous cannulation. It is this aspect of role development that I shall be concentrating on in this chapter. Although the individual nurse practitioner projects had been funded through the junior doctors' hours initiative, no additional money had been made available in order for ward-based staff to undertake extra duties.

I began the research with, what I considered to be, well-founded reasons for anticipating an increased need for negotiation and associated inter-occupational tension at the medical–nursing interface. The issue of boundary realignment between medicine and nursing was certainly a hot topic in the professional and policy media at this time. For example, on 15 October 1994 *The Guardian* examined 'The Sacking of Sister Pat' (Cook 1994), the case of a neurology sister dismissed by Plymouth Hospitals NHS Trust for making out a prescription for medication that was not signed by a doctor. The 'Pat Cooksley affair' was closely followed by the case of 'the appendix nurse', Valerie Tomlinson, a theatre sister who, under medical instruction, removed a patient's appendix. The *Nursing Standard* on 18 January 1995, in an editorial expressing surprise at the public outcry and media furore over the Tomlinson story, claimed that '[h]uge numbers of nurses are now undertaking duties which doctors used to perform' (Casey 1995a). Only six months later (19 July 1995), however, the title of the editorial conceded that 'Often "doctor job" (sic) have been thrust upon nursing and have added little to the enhancement of nursing practice' (Casey 1995b). That disagreements existed as to the appropriate allocation of medical and nursing work appeared to be confirmed elsewhere. For example, a survey study of nurses, junior doctors, and support workers undertaken in another part of the country prior to the research had revealed rank-and-file staff to be deeply ambivalent about the bracketing of nursing role developments with the junior doctors' hours initiative (Allen and Hughes 1993; Allen *et al.* 1993). Furthermore, Walby *et al.* (1994), in an extensive interview study of nursing and medicine in the changing health service, devote a whole chapter to exploring boundary conflicts between doctors and nurses.

The picture at Woodlands, however, was rather different from the one I had anticipated. As with the nurse–support worker interface, what I discovered was a combination of sustained negotiation and jurisdictional dispute in hospital management arenas, whereas at ward level, a realignment of doctors' and nurses' work roles appeared to be taking place with minimal negotiative effort and little explicit conflict – despite the ambivalence to the changes expressed by front-line staff. As with

Chapter 5, in order to provide the reader with a sense of the local policy context, I begin my examination of the empirical material with an analysis of the processes through which senior clinicians in the study site negotiated changes in the medical–nursing interface. Once again I will be drawing on the concept of 'boundary-work' (Gieryn 1983, 1991) as a way of understanding these negotiation processes.

Accomplishing policy change: the 'boundary-work' of medical and nurse managers

Nurse managers at Woodlands expressed uncertainty about changes in the nursing–medical boundary. Although they supported the principle of nursing role development, they felt that this should be patient-led and were concerned that in practice, shifts in nursing jurisdiction had become irrevocably linked with the junior doctors' hours initiative. Privately a number admitted that nurses were probably being 'dumped on' by the medical profession and hinted that the UKCC, in issuing its new guidelines on nurses' scope of professional practice, was in collusion with the government. Nevertheless, they recognized that junior doctors' hours had a high political profile and reasoned that it was preferable for nurses to expand their scope of practice than to allow another category of worker into the division of labour, which would further fragment patient care.[1]

The senior medical staff were happy to devolve certain technical tasks to nurses – intravenous antibiotic administration, venepuncture, ECGs, cannulation, and male urinary catheterization – although several expressed the view that it was important that doctors did not lose these skills. Where the tasks concerned came closer to the focal tasks of medicine – such as taking patient histories – they were rather more equivocal. Some indicated that they believed nursing staff had the skills to undertake this work in a limited sense provided they worked within clearly defined protocols. Others expressed the view that this entailed nurses making diagnoses, which was a responsibility that most doctors (and also nurses) believed should remain with medical staff.

> *I think diagnosis is likely always to remain the domain of the doctor.*
>
> (Consultant)

Taking control

Despite their reservations about its linkage with junior doctors' hours it was nurse managers who had taken control of the implementation of nursing role development. It seems that the nurse managers were galvanized into action by the fear that their medical colleagues would take control over the process, and, as such, their actions may be seen as an example of boundary-work.

> *There was almost like a splinter group of the medical staff and they were going to be writing the protocols for us which was one of the big pressures for the nursing staff to get their act together and to produce these packages and things because otherwise it would have been imposed on us from the medics. It's been a hell of a struggle getting all the paperwork sorted out but we didn't want someone else setting it up for us. We wanted to do everything ourselves.*
>
> (Nurse Manager)

In managing the process of boundary realignment, nurse managers and other senior nurses in the organization had developed a number of self-directed learning packages that staff had to complete and then sign to indicate that they were competent. At the time of the research this approach seemed at odds with the UKCC guidance on nurses' scope of practice, which had abolished the need for extended role certification. On reflection, however, I suggest that faced with the prospect of protocols being written for nurses by medical staff, the action of nurse managers may be understood as an important piece of 'boundary-work'. Control of education and training is vital in retaining professional jurisdiction (Jamous and Peloille 1970; Abbott 1988) and historically, nursing's professional project has been hamstrung by the difficulties in gaining control of the education and training of practitioners (Dingwall *et al.* 1988; Rafferty 1996). By insisting on taking charge of the education and training of nurses for role developments, the nurse managers were asserting the autonomy of nursing and resisting coming under the control of the medical profession.

Establishing expertise

In developing the learning packages, the nurse managers emphasized the need for ward staff to have an adequate knowledge-base to undertake devolved work. At one level this reflected risk management and litigation concerns, at another, it may also be seen as a further example of demarcatory processes. The following extract is taken from a meeting of senior nurses charged with responsibility for implementing nursing role developments at Woodlands. Two of the group members have expressed concern that the training packages were in danger of becoming bureaucratized.

NURSE MANAGER: I take these points that Simon and Felicity
    made about it – we're being in danger of it becoming a bit
    cumbersome – but I mean what I would want to say is that the
    fact that the doctors and phlebotomists aren't trained how to do
    it doesn't make it right does it?
NURSE PRACTITIONER [FELICITY]: No.
NURSE MANAGER: I mean surely we ought to be putting
    ourselves in a better position than that.
WARD MANAGER [SIMON]: I agree with you.

(Meeting)

By ensuring that practitioners had the underpinning knowledge to
support the changes in their role, senior nurses were establishing an
important boundary marker, which they felt differentiated nurses from
the 'see one, do one, teach one' training of medical staff, and from other
workers – such as phlebotomists and operating department assistants –
who were also being trained at Woodlands and in other hospitals in the
country to undertake similar activities. Moreover, as textual representa-
tions of nursing knowledge, the learning packages may also be understood as important boundary signifiers in the social production of nursing
jurisdiction in the study site, which differentiated the nursing contribution from that of lower-level occupational groups and junior doctors.

Nurses' attempts to establish expertise were ridiculed by senior
medical staff, however, who – in undertaking 'boundary-work' of their
own – claimed that the detailed knowledge included in the training packages was superfluous. The following extracts begin with comments which
were made in a letter to the Director of Medicine by a consultant surgeon.

re. Scope of Professional Practice – Flushing of Central Lines
[...]
I find this document exceedingly complex and probably over
comprehensive for the needs of nursing staff who may be
required to flush a central line. In fact, it is so complex that I
myself am unable to answer some of the questions required of
the nursing staff, and I suspect that the majority of the medical
staff within the hospital would also be unable to satisfactorily
complete the questions. I feel that if the protocol is to be
adopted within the hospital, and I myself am unable to comply
with it, then I must regard myself as being unsuitable for the
insertion, let alone the flushing of central lines (sic). On this
basis I would suggest that I am no longer a suitable person for
the insertion of these lines, including of course Hickman and

129

other central lines. I would therefore suggest that we no longer use central lines within this hospital.

(Document – internal communication)

This theme was also echoed in the interview data.

[It's] crazy – for what is a practical procedure with some theory behind it, actually putting it into a context where the theory is totally out-stripping the practical nature that it's intended for. And nurses are practical people at the end of the day.

(Consultant)

They've produced a manual! [...] all they needed was to spend an afternoon in theatre. If someone needs two hourly turns they order her a special bed because there's a tissue viability nurse.

(Consultant)

There are clear parallels here with features of the 'boundary-work' in which nurse managers engaged in accomplishing the nurse–support worker interface (Chapter 5). To recapitulate briefly, we noted that the status of a given activity is not fixed and, in the context of boundary disputes, may be contested. One important dimension of the contested nature of an area of work is the relative proportion of indeterminate and technical skills required to perform the tasks concerned (Jamous and Peloille 1970). A higher margin of indeterminate work provides a stronger basis for maintaining jurisdictional control. The 'boundary-work' of the senior medical staff presented here can be seen as micro-political processes of this kind, that is, as an attempt to recast nurses in the subordinate role of technician in the face of their more elevated claims.

Identity work

The contested nature of activities at the medical–nursing interface was also evident in clinical managers' accounts of boundary realignment in which medical and nursing staff constituted the task area in quite different ways. Doctors typically down-graded the tasks that were being devolved to nursing, emphasizing their repetitive, practical nature and their relative safety.

It is not difficult to put in a cannula and the more that you do the better at it you get.

(Consultant)

I mean the specific skills could be taught to anybody who's reasonably conscientious, careful and sensible.

(Consultant)

[A] lot of what the juniors were doing were these repetitive tasks which were no good for their educational training [...] nurses are good at doing repetitive tasks [laughs]. So you know, to be able to get nurses to do the tasks that were indicated like IV drugs, catheters, [...] and taking blood, giving intravenous injections was fine – the so-called drudgery.

(Consultant)

Nurse managers' accounts, on the other hand, were permeated with the rhetoric of holism. This was a useful discursive device through which they were able to bring the nurse–patient relationship into play so as to construct a higher margin of indeterminacy around the task area and fabricate a distinctive approach to patient care.

Sarah [Nurse Practitioner] said that [...] [The doctors] just want to shove an IV in. They don't think about the patient as a whole.

[Y]ou don't only need the skills to cannulate you need the skills to look at the patient.

(Senior Nurse)

[W]e're not developing our skills just to take off the menial jobs from the doctors, [...] we're doing it because we want to and because it's more holistic individualized patient care.

(Senior Nurse)

I have a lot of excitement about *The Scope* because I think for nursing it's, nurses are in an ideal position to give more holistic care, not tasks. You know you ring the doctor up and it doesn't matter who the doctor is but he'll come along and do the IVs for you. He might never have seen that patient. But if a nurse has got a relationship and understanding with the patient and she spends a bit of time giving an IV then there's a lot of communication and relationship-building going on there.

(Interview – Nurse Manager)

At one level, the field actors' accounts may be understood as evidence of the broader micro-politics at work in the study site over the meaning and value of activities situated at the medical–nursing interface. At another level, however, these data arise in the interview context and so can also be understood in terms of the locally situated 'identity work' they are rhetorically assembled to perform. The concept of 'identity work' is widely used in the literature to refer to the impression management activities (Goffman 1959) in which individuals engage to accomplish a particular type of personal identity. Snow and Anderson (1987) suggest that the social construction of identity can entail management of physical settings and props, attention to personal appearance (see, for example, Phelan and Hunt 1998), selective association with individuals and/or groups, as well as the narrative construction of particular identities (see, for example, Snow and Anderson 1987; Cohan 1997; Antaki and Widdicombe 1998; Rosenfeld 1999). Hunt and Benford (1994) argue that identity talk is a 'discourse that reflects actors' perceptions of a social order and is based on interpretations of current situations, themselves and others' (p. 492).

By constituting the nature of these devolved activities in such different ways, I suggest that the medical and nursing managers were attempting to construct accounts of shifts in the division of labour that were consistent with their respective occupational identities and their perceptions of the position of nursing and medicine within it. Doctors rhetorically constituted the task area so as to subordinate the nursing contribution to that of a technician, whereas nurses explicitly resisted the charge that they were unwilling recipients of doctors' dirty work and emphasized their distinctive professional contribution to care and the indeterminacy involved in the production process. The interactional work being done here relates to the identification of the nursing and medical managers with their respective clinical occupations and their associated professional rhetoric and, as such, this occupational identity work may be considered a variant of boundary-work.

Unlike the management arena in which changes in the medical–nursing boundary were being explicitly negotiated and contested, however, grass-roots workers were accomplishing boundary realignment with little overt conflict and minimal negotiative effort. It is to this negotiative arena that I now wish to turn.

Accomplishing the medical–nursing boundary on the wards

The view from the front-line

Ward nurses described the incorporation of doctor-devolved activities into their work as double-edged. Employing a mixture of professional and management discourses, they identified advantages for patient care but also expressed concern that further expansion of their jurisdiction would make it even more difficult for them to create space to undertake sustained patient contact work, which they regarded as a central reward of the job.

> *Part of me wants to do it and part of me feels that if I do that then it's taking me away from the patients again.*
>
> (Staff Nurse)

> *I think that sometimes it takes us away from the simple idea of what a nurse is for and what the patient thinks we're for. I think it's a good idea when you haven't got the doctor and there's an IV to be given and you can't get one and the nurse can give it on time.*
>
> (Staff Nurse)

Like their senior colleagues, the junior doctors in this study were more than happy for nurses to take over what they regarded as low status menial activities, but many were clear that certain of these were essential medical skills that they themselves did not want to lose.

> *Taking blood and putting in cannulas. Especially putting in cannulas. I think that's very important. I think it is a vital skill that doctors should have really.*
>
> (HO)

Doctors were divided as to whether expanded role activities should be shared with nursing staff or permanently devolved, whereas most of the nurses believed tasks should be shared with medical staff and undertaken according to the exigencies of the work. But despite the equivocality of ward-based staff about their changing inter-occupational boundaries my field observations revealed that jurisdictional shifts were managed with minimal negotiation and little explicit conflict.

A non-negotiated order?

When I asked them how they managed the boundaries of their work in daily practice, the nurses emphasized their jurisdictional control. They insisted that their priority was nursing care; if busy, they expected to negotiate the allocation of work with medical staff.

DA: When do you decide whether you will do these things rather than the doctor?

133

STAFF NURSE: Whether I'm busy or not. Nursing comes first
and it's my registration on the line. I'm here to do nursing and
the patients perceive that to be my role.

These accounts are clearly consistent with the UKCC's guidance on
nurses' scope of practice (UKCC 1992), which states that role expansion should not lead to the inappropriate delegation of 'nursing care'.
My observations suggested that in practice, however, this was more the
case of a shift in the nurse–doctor boundary rather than a negotiated
domain of work. Despite their reservations about role expansion and
their commitment to nursing care activities, those nurses who had the
skills to undertake doctor-devolved tasks did so regardless of their other
work pressures.

One way of interpreting this discrepancy between nurses' claims and
their observed practice, is as a reflection of their efforts to demonstrate
their continuing control over their work boundaries so as to accomplish
a competent professional performance. Contemporary nursing ideology
emphasizes nurses' autonomous practitioner status. By insisting they
had choices about whether to undertake doctor-devolved work, the
nurses in this study may have been attempting to resist the charge that
they were being 'dumped on' by the medical profession wishing to
discard their 'dirty work'. In other words they were doing identity work.
Yet, although it clearly jarred with nurses' professional identities,
carrying out doctor-devolved activities was a perfectly rational response
to the constraints of the work context.

I have shown in previous chapters that the turbulence of the
hospital environment fashions nursing jurisdiction in complex ways.
In order to comprehend why nurses constituted the boundaries of their
work in the shape that they did, and thus how the changing division of
labour between nurses and doctors was accomplished with minimal
negotiation and little explicit conflict, we need to focus on two key
features of the work setting: the respective transience and permanence
of nursing and medical staff and the fragmented temporal–spatial
organization of medical and nursing work. As with the support worker
boundary, the strategies staff employed in managing these characteristics of the work setting meant that the non-negotiated blurring of
medical and nursing jurisdiction was actually a normal characteristic
of nurses' routine practice. I suggest that when it is recognized that
non-negotiated boundary-blurring was a taken-for-granted feature of
nursing work, then the lack of inter-occupational negotiation and overt
conflict relating to policy-driven shifts in the hospital division of
labour becomes understandable.

Transience and permanence

The hospital drew heavily on the immediate community for its non-medical staff. Most of the nurses had trained locally and staff turnover was low. Compared with the nurses, junior doctors were transient members of the ward team. HOs rotated as frequently as every 3 months, SHOs every 6 months, with registrars staying in post for up to a year. Conversely, few of the junior doctors were local; many had come from overseas and, like the doctors in Hughes' (1988) study of work in accident and emergency, their transient status was exacerbated by cultural difference and lack of familiarity with the UK health system.

Weber (1970) has indicated that, bureaucrats may have considerable power over political incumbents, as a result, in part, of their permanence within the political bureaucracy, contrasted to public officials, who are replaced more frequently. Low ranking officials become familiar with the organization, its rules and operation, which gives them power over the new political incumbent (Lipsky 1980). The ethnographic literature suggests that the relative permanency of nursing staff can augment their influence vis-à-vis doctors (Mumford 1970; Bucher and Stelling 1977; Myers 1979; Roth and Douglas 1983; Haas and Shaffir 1987; Hughes 1988). Where turnover of nurses is rapid, however, their influence is likely to be significantly compromised (Dingwall *et al.* 1983).

In this study, the permanence of nurses and the transience of medical staff, created discontinuities of experience and status. Nurses wielded considerable influence. Doctors relied on them for guidance on details of local protocols and aspects of ward practice as well as for the location of materials and equipment.

STAFF GRADE DOCTOR: What do I have to write on here?

STAFF NURSE: Just write 'Dextrose powder for glucose tolerance'.

STAFF GRADE DOCTOR: Do I need to fill in a special form or do you just carry it out?

STAFF NURSE: We just do it.

STAFF GRADE DOCTOR: [to DA] I don't think I am the best candidate to study because I am new to the NHS and I ask more questions than I should.

STAFF NURSE: Did you just want a chest X-ray on that lady?

HO: And bloods.

135

STAFF NURSE: A and E [accident and emergency] did bloods for you.
HO: Did they? They didn't write it down.
STAFF NURSE: Yes. She came down with two packages and I noticed you'd not done an X-ray [completed a request form]. I've done that for you.

Nurses were often more knowledgeable than doctors about aspects of the ward speciality and this enabled them to influence treatment decisions.

STAFF NURSE: She's on pre-meal BMs [blood sugar monitoring].
SENIOR SISTER: They [the doctors] said they wanted pre-meal and post-meal! I said 'We don't do that'! [Laughter]
(Handover)

Nurses frequently questioned junior doctors' drug prescriptions if they differed from the standard medication regimes with which they were familiar.

STAFF NURSE: This has been written as a PRN [as required] MST.
HO: It seems fair enough?
STAFF NURSE: It's a bit silly isn't it? Can't it be Oromorph instead. It's only for – she's having debridement of her shoulder tomorrow.
The house officer alters the kardex.

STAFF NURSE: [to HO] I just want to query this Erythromycin. Do you want it just once a day? It's usually twice a day.
HO changes the prescription.

Nurses routinely requested specific drug prescriptions for patients and were rarely questioned by medical staff.

Staff Nurse goes to HO with a pile of drugs kardexes and hands HO a chart.
STAFF NURSE: Can you just prescribe Paracetamol there for us?
HO: Ah hhh. [Writes on the drugs chart].
STAFF NURSE [HANDING HO ANOTHER CHART]: This lady's one of ours. For some reason she's got two drug kardexes and there's Pethidine on both.
HO: Is she in pain? [Looks at charts]

STAFF NURSE: She's on Dihydrocodeine [points to chart] and that needs writing up properly as well. Mega constipation!
HO: Dr Anwar – what is he thinking of? [Crosses out some of the prescribed times for administration].
STAFF NURSE [hands HO another drug chart]: And this is the last one. Can you write her up for PRN nebulisers? She's very breathless.
HO: [HO writes on chart and hands it back] There you are.

The informal prescribing power of nursing staff is revealed by the observation that nurses referred to doctors as 'writing up' drugs rather than prescribing them. Doctors, for their part, freely acknowledged the skills and influence of nursing staff.

> [A] nursing sister who's been on a unit for years knows far more than I do. We learn molecules and chemical biology in our training. You don't get the clinical feel until much later.
>
> (Registrar)

> To be realistic about it, most of it is what they [junior doctors] learn themselves from the nursing staff by being told 'This is what happens on the ward. This is how to do things. This is what the consultant expects. This is what is required.'
>
> (Consultant)

These findings are consistent with those of recent ethnographic studies (Hughes 1988; Stein *et al*. 1990; Porter 1991, 1995; Svensson 1996; Wicks 1998), which indicate that much contemporary nurse–doctor interaction goes beyond the passive influence attempts described by Stein (1967) in his account of the doctor–nurse game. Moreover, it is clear that the relative permanence of nurses augmented their influence over key aspects of medical practice and education, which resulted in a modification of the traditional division of nursing and medical knowledge and expertise. In order to understand how this contributed to the non-negotiated blurring of the technical division of labour between nursing and medical staff, we need to analyse its interactive effects with a second feature of medical and nursing work: its fragmented temporal–spatial organization.

The temporal–spatial organization of nursing and medical work
Twenty-four-hour medical and nursing coverage was provided 365 days a year but accomplished in rather different ways. Patient care was

137

provided by nursing and support staff via a three-shift system, whereas junior doctors routinely worked office hours, Monday to Friday. Outside normal working hours medical cover was provided by the on-call team. Medical and nursing work also had a different spatial organization. Nurses were ward-based but the work of junior doctors took them to other wards and departments.

The difference in the temporal–spatial organization of medical and nursing work was most marked outside normal hours when doctors were on-call. The on-call period was for 24 hours and ran from 9 a.m. The on-call team were responsible for all admissions in their particular directorate[2] and emergency ward cover. On weekdays, ward cover did not commence until 5 p.m., but at the weekend and on public holidays the on-call team were responsible for ward work for the full 24-hour period. The introduction of an Admissions Unit[3] meant that doctors spent little sustained time on the wards during the on-call period.

The different temporal–spatial organization of medical and nursing work created rather different perspectives and priorities, which were a source of strain. Nurses' sights were focused on the needs of the patients on their wards, whereas doctors were concerned with the whole directorate and new admissions. Doctors tried to organize their work so that they attended to patients in order of clinical priority but were also concerned to minimize unnecessary 'leg work' as they moved between different departments throughout the hospital. Nurses were ever-conscious of the constraints of external organizational timetables and considerable nursing effort went into co-ordinating patient care activities and ensuring that treatments were carried out according to schedule. Moreover, it was nurses who were directly confronted with the distress of patients and/or relatives.

Strains

In their study of nursing and medicine in the UK, Walby *et al.* (1994) argue that nearly half the points of conflict they identified between doctors and nurses could be traced to the different spatial and geographic organization of nursing and medical work. These strains are often reflected in tensions over the bleep system. A common nursing complaint at Woodlands was the difficulty they had in getting doctors to attend the ward. Owing to their proximity to the patient, nurses have a key role in co-ordinating patient care and protecting them from the organizational turbulence of the hospital setting. When doctors were unavailable this greatly increased the burdens on nursing staff. Equally, however, on-call doctors frequently worked under immense pressures and quickly became irritated when their work was constantly inter-rupted by the bleep. Although the junior doctors felt that other members of the health care team did not understand the on-call experi-ence, nurses' frustration with their medical colleagues' absence from the wards was mediated by their sympathy for the burdens doctors faced.

The temporal–spatial ordering of medical and nursing work creates a second, related tension, which mirrors those described by Whyte (1979) in his study of restaurant work. Whyte argues that a central problem of the large restaurant is to tie together its line of authority with the rela-tions that arise along its flow of work. In a restaurant, the flow of work usually originates with the customer and is passed to the waitresses who then have to initiate the work of higher status countermen or barmen. Whyte proposes that relations among individuals along the flow of work will run more smoothly when those of higher status are in a position to initiate work for those of lower status in the organization, and conversely, that friction will be observed more often when lower status individuals seek to initiate the work of those with higher status. According to Whyte, a number of strategies are developed in restaurants – either consciously or unconsciously – to cut down waitresses' origina-tion of action for higher status staff. For example, the rule that orders must be written cuts down interaction, although not always enough to eliminate friction.

Similar problems arise in relation to doctors and nurses. Although the nurses were prepared to negotiate with individual doctors in a direct way about certain aspects of patient treatment, they were also clearly oriented to medicine's superordinate status within the formal organiza-tion. This created strains because owing to the temporal–spatial ordering of their respective activities, it was nurses who initiated much of medical work.

Staff at the point of service delivery employed a number of strategies to manage these tensions. For example, nurses expended considerable effort organizing doctors' work; tasks were saved up, rather than the doctor being bleeped for every single problem as it occurred. Another tactic was to anticipate patient requirements and ensure that doctors had prescribed 'PRN' (as required) medications so that nurses could respond to patient need without having to contact the doctor. One HO had developed the practice of signing blank dietician referral forms so that they were available when nurses required them. By far the most important way in which these strains were managed, however, was by nurses routinely undertaking a whole range of activities that fell outside their formal jurisdiction.

Managing the strains – blurring the nurse–doctor boundary

In one sense, of course, some blurring of the medical–nursing boundary is unavoidable. This reflects the impossibility of sustaining a formal division of labour in which doctors diagnose and nurses merely observe. At a fairly mundane level, out of the wealth of information nurses gather about their patients they have to decide what is medically relevant (Gamarnikow 1991). Just as nurses' 'knowing' of the patient is filtered through the interpretative lens of support workers, the medical 'gaze' (Foucault 1976) is articulated through and mediated by nursing practice (Gamarnikow 1991). I have called this *de facto* boundary-blurring. Nurses also undertook *purposive* boundary-blurring work, however, of which I have identified five sub-types.

Continuity-oriented boundary-blurring was undertaken in order to ensure patient treatment was not interrupted. Most common was the example of nurses 'prescribing' additional intravenous fluids when the doctor was unavailable to amend the chart.

> I observed Glenda [staff nurse] putting up a bag of IV saline on a patient for whom it was not prescribed. She was discussing the matter with the senior sister who made the final decision that Glenda should put the bag up. She said that Glenda should put the IV up and that it could always come down if it wasn't right. It was clear that the senior sister was slightly uneasy about the fact that I was at the desk and observing this.

Nursing staff also informally blurred nursing and medical jurisdiction to ensure co-ordination of the work. This *articulation-oriented* boundary-blurring occurred when nurses requested standard blood tests so they were ready for the phlebotomist, and tests were carried out on time. Moreover, investigations and referrals were frequently initiated by staff on the basis of their own judgement (*judgemental* boundary-blurring), for instance, when nurses requested blood tests if they thought patients looked anaemic.

> STAFF NURSE: She looked a bit anaemic so I found an HB form! [she'd written one out].

> Staff nurse said that she would fill in the blood forms and specimen forms if she was not busy. She said, 'If I've been with the doctor seeing a difficult patient then I will do the forms if I'm not too busy.' She told me 'they were clamping down on the 'PPs' now – you shouldn't do it. So now we just make a

scrawl.' Staff Nurse told me that they would accept a form from the Nurse Practitioner 'So we can put that on it if we get stuck. But if we didn't do it then they wouldn't get done.'

Rule-oriented boundary-blurring occurred when nurses worked in the spirit of one rule even if this meant breaking another. Nurses routinely gave saline flushes after the administration of intravenous antibiotics even if it was not prescribed. Here, nurses were honouring the hospital policy that recommended saline flushes to follow intravenous antibiotics, although they were prohibited from prescribing medications. It was also relatively common practice for nurses to administer unprescribed drugs and request the doctor to prescribe them later. Nurses justified this *lay-oriented* boundary-blurring on the basis of the action patient, would have taken, had they been at home.

> I saw a note for drugs to be written up 'Lactulose please'. The junior sister 'confessed' to me that on the drugs round she had given a patient Lactulose and was going to get the doctors to write it up later. She said, 'Actually I've been a bit naughty I've given him some Lactulose and I'll get Andrew [SHO] to write it up later.'

Yet nurses had not simply incorporated this work into their everyday practice. When doctors were present on the ward, nursing staff adhered to hospital policy and asked the doctor to carry out these tasks. It was also more common for experienced nurses to blur occupational boundaries than junior staff. Indeed I observed nurses asking their senior colleagues to do their boundary-blurring work for them. In addition, nurses were most likely to break the rules for doctors they trusted.

> If you were going to break the rules you'd always do it for someone that you trusted than someone you didn't.
>
> (Staff Nurse)

Interestingly, there was little purposive boundary-blurring at night. This was surprising: the ethnographic literature (Roth and Douglas 1983; Porter 1995) indicates that during the night-shift nurses carry out many duties they do not do during the day in order to give the on-call physician a rest. There seemed to be a number of possible explanations for the dearth of informal boundary-blurring on the night-shift at Woodlands. First, the working environment at night was not as turbulent as it was during the day and ward nurses were less preoccupied with co-ordination activities. Second, night staff did not have established relationships with medical staff. With the opening of the admissions Unit, doctors no longer spent prolonged periods on the wards dealing with new patient admissions. Third, nursing care at night was provided by a separate night staff that had its own social order. All of the night nurses I spoke to were quite clear that they would not give unprescribed drugs to patients. Many justified their position by recounting the same 'moral tale'.

> *I heard on the grapevine. She gave Temazepam and asked the doctor to write it up later, which she would have done, but somebody told a tale and she was sacked for prescribing.*
>
> (Staff Nurse)

A further interesting anomaly is that throughout the fieldwork period, a recurring feature in nurses', support workers' and doctors' accounts was their concern with risk management and issues of litigation and yet this does not appear to have stopped them from breaking organizational rules in order to accomplish the work. One possible explanation for this is that boundary-blurring was such a taken-for-granted feature of normal practice that staff did not routinely reflect upon its implications.

Making sense of nurses' non-negotiated boundary-blurring

The discrepancy between nurses' accounts of their work and their actual practice suggested that their boundary-blurring clearly strained their professional identities. Furthermore, as we have seen, it led them to break hospital rules and, in certain instances, violate statutory jurisdictional boundaries. Notwithstanding these considerations, however, it undoubtedly benefited patients. As a result of nurses' flexible working practices, patients received symptom relief when they needed it, diagnostic investigations were carried out on time and treatment was continued without interruption. As such, nurses' flexible working practices constituted a vital organizational glue that made an important contribution to clinical effectiveness (Allen and Lyne 1997) and acted as an antidote to the centrifugal effects of the modern hospital setting. Doctors recognized the skills of nursing staff and were grateful when nurses were prepared to employ those skills in ways that eased their burden of work.

HO: Diane on geriatrics is brill. She really sticks her neck out. She's really good.

DA: In what sense?

HO: Well, she prescribes things say like Maxolon. I get there and she says she's done it.

STAFF NURSE: She's had some indigestion, burning pain and I gave her some Malox.

HO: Thank you for being so keen. I was once bleeped at six in the morning to give some Malox!'

Given the informal influence nurses wielded over treatment decisions, it was only a small step to take this further and do the work themselves when the situation demanded it. Furthermore, given the strains arising from the fragmented temporal organization of their work and the disjuncture between the flow of work and their orientation to formal organizational hierarchies, it was often easier and less time-consuming for nurses to undertake the work than it was to try and negotiate with the doctor to do it.

> You can bleep the doctor and wait for six hours or do it yourself!
>
> (Staff Nurse)

Staff Nurse said he was eager to extend his skills rather than having to spend time trying to get the doctor to do these things he could just do it himself.

> It's not ideal because I am guilty of doing things I shouldn't do. I mean I do blood forms and things like that even though I know I shouldn't. Because it's an easier life and I know things are going to get done. In theory yes it should be well-defined but practically it's not always possible. I'm guilty on that really.
>
> (Junior Sister)

> [Y]ou know what they [doctors] are willing to do and the hassle it is to get them to do the little menial jobs. It's just not worth the hassle sometimes. It's just easier to get it done and get on with it and say 'Right this is the result do something with it.'
>
> (Staff Nurse)

It was nurses, moreover, who were in the firing line if patients were waiting on doctors.

STAFF NURSE: The thing is this is really the doctors' work but if we didn't do this then the doctors wouldn't do it and TTOs [medications to take home] aren't written up and then it comes back on us doesn't it when the patients get cross and they can't go home.

This illustrates the point made by Strauss (1978), that members' perceived options are important in understanding the decision of whether to embark upon negotiations or not.

Critics have suggested that extended roles erode nurses' claim to autonomous practitioner status by bringing the occupation under medical control (Tomich 1978). On the wards, however, nurses' boundary-blurring actually gave them greater local autonomy over their work, improved patient care, and had the additional advantage of avoiding inter-personal tension. Nurses' non-negotiated boundary-blurring clearly made sense within the work context. Nevertheless, these findings raise important questions about the constraints within which nurses worked, which made non-negotiated boundary-blurring their easiest option and the implications that this had for their professional identities. As we have seen, many of the staff in this study expressed dissatisfaction with the content and shape of their work. This is a complex issue that relates to a number of the boundaries examined in this book, and one I will return to in Chapter 9.

8

THE NURSE–PATIENT
BOUNDARY

Given my substantive focus thus far, the inclusion of a chapter on nurses and patients might seem a surprising addition to this book. Yet, as with its internal division of labour and its relationships with other occupational groups, nursing jurisdiction is, to a considerable extent, shaped by the boundary of its work with that of patients and this, like other interfaces within the wider societal division of labour, is also affected by historical and political factors.

Since the rise of organized medicine at the beginning of the twentieth century, what is known as an 'acute-care' philosophy has underpinned the medical–nursing care in hospital settings. This was reflected in the classic picture of the 'sick role' described by Parsons (1951) of an acutely ill person, temporarily passive and acquiescent, being treated by an active physician and carers (Strauss *et al.* 1985). Because the lay–professional encounter was founded on an asymmetry of expertise, it was necessary for the patient to trust the professionals and co-operate with them in order to benefit from their services, or so it was argued. While vestiges of this orthodoxy clearly remain, current thinking about the role of the patient is centred on a model of the lay public as knowledgeable partners in health care. Both within nursing and within the wider health policy arena, efforts are being made to move towards more active models of care based on shared decision-making and greater user control.

This change in thinking has been shaped by a number of considerations. First, the late 1960s and early 1970s saw the emergence of a number of critiques of modern medicine that questioned its achievements (McKeown 1965), and suggested that it could even be having a deleterious effect on society, for example, by eroding people's ability to deal with their own problems (Illich 1976). The structural inequalities that characterized the professional–patient relationship had hitherto been described in fairly benign terms, but by the 1960s the study of professions had acquired a more critical edge. Earlier scholars were accused of naively accepting the ideology and rhetoric of the established professions. Rather than serving disembodied social needs, professions imposed their own definition of needs on clients and were thus a form of social control, it was claimed (Johnson 1967; Freidson 1970a,b; Larson 1977). Freidson (1970a,b) went so far as to suggest that 'medical dominance' was the analytic key to the inadequacies of the health service. The bureaucratic, paternalistic and impersonal nature of health care provision was the product of a system in which the doctor was the designated expert and all other opinions (including lay ones) were subordinate. Because the domination of medicine was total, Freidson argued, it not only affected the doctor-patient relationship but it also shaped the nature of the relations between other health professionals and patients, including nurses. Many of the empirical studies spawned by this more critical body of work focused on issues of information and communication. In particular, attention was directed at the failure of members of the medical profession to inform patients about their condition and treatment. Critics argued that not only was the withholding of information a source of considerable distress to patients, but it was also a further way in which the profession of medicine consolidated its power (Roth 1963; Glaser and Strauss 1965; Davis 1972; Quint 1972; McIntosh 1977).

Second, as a result of public health improvements and developments in medical technology there has been a shift from acute illness to the dominance of chronic conditions that require continuing management. The long-term nature of chronic diseases makes lay participation particularly appropriate, given that continuing care is needed. The management of chronic disease is often complex, requiring medications, special diets, exercise regimes and monitoring and assessment of the condition. Sufferers develop particular kinds of skills and knowledge derived from their daily experience of living with their condition and yet, in the past, they have been expected to delegate this responsibility to professional staff on admission to hospital. In recent years there has been an increase in the number of support groups focused on a specific disease or condition that can be an important source of practical help and emotional support for sufferers and their families.

Finally, there has been long-standing concern about the escalating costs of health provision, which has had implications for the lay–professional boundary in a number of respects. First, it has fuelled the desire of policy makers to augment the power of service users to counter that of the health professions. Second, it has focused attention on the potentially preventable demands placed on the Service. Third, it has resulted in changes in thinking about state involvement in welfare provision.

In the UK these trends have led to attempts to reshape the role of lay people in health care in two important ways. First, efforts have been made to change the nature of the lay–professional relationship by redressing the traditional power imbalance between service users and health care professionals. This was manifested in the rise of consumerism in the health care sector, which was evident in the Griffiths Report and later consolidated in the 1990 NHS and Community Care Act. Purchasers and providers are now required to take 'consumer' views into account when developing services and individual patients are expected to secure their rights under a contractual model of social relations (Annandale 1998). The discourse may have changed under the current government – policy makers have discarded the vocabulary of the market, preferring, instead, to talk in terms of 'partnerships' with 'service users' – but the emphasis on lay involvement in health care is still very much in evidence. For example, the patient/carer perspective is one of six areas in the New National Performance Framework set out in the White Paper *The New NHS Modern and Dependable* (DH 1998a) and its Welsh counterpart – *Putting Patients First* (NHS Wales 1998) – refers to 'user involvement' in the definition of quality standards and clinical audit. Additionally, as part of its policy research programme, the Department of Health has also established an initiative related to the development of 'partnerships' with patients, carers and the public in health care decision-making (DH 1998c).

Although there has been much talk of the rights and entitlements of citizens in relation to lay participation, these developments have a second face that is focused on responsibilities and obligations. As Sayer (1996, cited by Webb, 1999) has pointed out, the rhetoric of 'empowerment' has been coupled with that of 'responsibilization'. Contemporary systems of welfare increasingly emphasize self-help in the management of health and illness. For example, it is now assumed that family or significant others will care for their dependent relatives. Considerable attention has also been given to individuals' responsibility for their health. The White Paper, *The Health of the Nation states:*

> We live in an age where many of the main causes of premature death and unnecessary disease are related to how we live our lives.

> (DH 1992: 2)

Accordingly, health promotion has become a central plank of policy in recent years, although under the incumbent Labour administration, the emphasis on individual responsibility has been tempered by a greater recognition of the socio-economic bases of ill health (see, for example, DH 1998b). Moreover, in addition to being instructed to lead healthy lives, we are now being explicitly encouraged to self-manage certain conditions (as evidenced by the availability of what were formerly 'prescription only medicines' through the pharmacist) as well as being trained in the appropriate use of health services.

Similar changes to the lay–professional boundary are also evident within nursing, although to what extent they are a reflection of wider societal trends or whether nursing has itself provided some of the impetus for these changes in thinking is difficult to assess. In recent years, professional discourses have brought about a reconstruction of the nursing function in which relationships with patients figure prominently. 'Patient participation' is now a central dimension of the nursing role. 'New nursing' ideology advocates participatory models of practice based on the active engagement of the client. Emphasis has been given to the need to provide adequate information and involve patients in the assessment of their needs and the planning, provision and evaluation of their care. Mindful of the dangers of fostering dependency, nursing care is designed to promote patient independence; teaching and health promotion are now also considered central to nurses' role. Moreover, contemporary nursing rhetoric underlines the importance of patients' subjective experience of their illness and its interaction with their daily lives. Nurses are now encouraged to develop close relationships with patients so that they can understand the meaning their illness has for them and to use this knowledge to jointly plan individually tailored programmes of care. Primary nursing is considered the ideal mode of work organization to facilitate participatory relationships of this kind.

While at one level, certainly, these developments within nursing may be interpreted as an attempt to improve the care given to patients, at another, they need also to be understood in the context of nursing's aspirations to professional status. Although the refashioning of the nurse–patient boundary is clearly unorthodox in terms of the traditional model of professionalism – because of their informed position professionals are conventionally regarded as more knowledgeable than clients and so clients do not, therefore, constitute a significant reference group – the crucial point is that alignment with the patient also legitimates the empowerment of nurses, vis-à-vis doctors. Exponents of 'new nursing' maintain that individually planned care and shared decision-making can only empower the patient if the carer has the power to enact those decisions.

> If the patient is to enjoy freedom of choice and the nurse is to
> be the agent of this choice, then the nurse also must be

empowered and have the freedom to make decisions as an
autonomous practitioner.

(Trnobranski 1994: 734)

Despite the widespread acceptance of the desirability of these changes
in the patient–professional boundary there is a surprising dearth of theorizing in this area. The literature contains a bewildering array of terms –
'patient participation', 'lay participation', 'user involvement', 'collaborative care', 'self-care', 'partnership', 'consumerism' – which are used
to mean different things by different people, often for different political
purposes. One thing that these terms all have in common, however, is
that they conflate those changes to the lay–professional boundary that
affects citizen's rights and to those that have implications for their
responsibilities. For example, much cited in nursing scholarship is
Brearley's (1990) review of patient participation. Having acknowledged
the problem of conceptual obfuscation in this area, Brearley adopts a
definition of participation proposed by Brownlea (1987), which
embraces decision-making, evaluation and consultation on the one
hand, and service delivery on the other:

> Participation means getting involved or being allowed to
> become involved in a decision-making process or the delivery
> of a service or the evaluation of a service, or even simply to
> become one of a number of people consulted on an issue or a
> matter.
>
> (Brearley 1990: 4, quoting Brownlea 1987)

A corollary of this failure to distinguish between these two aspects of
the lay–professional boundary has been an uncritical tendency both
within nursing and wider policy circles to assume that, at the level of the
individual certainly, increased 'participation' in health care brings with
it a concomitant increase in the power of the lay person vis-à-vis health
care providers. Furthermore, some of the tensions inherent in these basic
ideas with which health professionals and the lay public must grapple
have not been adequately addressed. For example, while the right side
of the equation underlines the importance of patient involvement in
decision-making and assessment of the quality of services, the flip side
emphasizes their responsibility for health maintenance, which, by impli-
cation, means compliance with medical edicts on healthy living and
disease management. Yet people may have very rational reasons for not
following medical advice. Lay knowledge is of a different order from
professional knowledge and, from the perspective of the sufferer it is

subtly superior (Macintyre and Oldman 1977). The patient's knowledge of his or her disease is rooted in his or her everyday life and his or her experience of illness, whereas the doctor works from objectified disease processes (Williams and Popay 1994). Service providers, for their part, are being expected to accommodate individual patient preferences in a climate of growing economic stringency, where their clinical practice is increasingly subject to external scrutiny and pressure towards standardization, and the fear of complaints and litigation looms large.

Given these considerations, I suggest that the division of labour framework developed in this book offers a potentially fruitful way of analysing these changes to the nurse–patient boundary. Rather than searching for a satisfactory definition of 'participation' or its synonyms, this approach involves a conceptualization of the patient as a co-worker (Stacey 1976; Hughes 1984; Strauss *et al.* 1985) in the provision of health care and consideration of the following questions: What kinds of work are carried out in sustaining health and coping with illness? Who does that work? How are activities negotiated between workers? What is the nature of the relationship between workers?

I suggest that Hughes' (1984) analytic distinction between the moral and technical division of labour, which was introduced in Chapter 2, offers a useful conceptual framework with which to examine the role and task dimensions of the nurse–patient boundary, both individually and in terms of their interrelations. Moreover, it permits consideration of the nature of the relationship between patients and all health care workers, including those who do not fit the archetype of profession. As Hughes (1984) and Stacey (1976) have pointed out, although the patient is a worker in the health care division of labour, the fact that they are also the work object and the service object of others colours the nature of their interactions.

Changes in the 'technical division of labour' between nurses and patients

Within sociology, there has been a burgeoning literature on lay health care behaviours of varying kinds in recent years (see, for example, Macintyre and Oldman 1977; Anderson and Bury 1988; Murphy 1999; Williams 2000). But explicit recognition of the health care *work* performed by patients is associated mainly with the writings of Strauss *et al.* (1985), although Hughes also includes the patient in the division of labour in health care (1984: 308) and Goffman's (1961) work has shown that even in the most oppressed conditions the patient is not just a passive recipient of care (Stacey 1976). More recently Stacey (1976, 1992) has also underlined the importance of conceptualizing the patient as a health worker.

According to Strauss *et al.* patients may be immersed in the ward division of labour in different ways. First, staff expect patients to work (whether or not it is actually called work): reluctant patients are subject to sanctions. Second, patients are sometimes invited into the division of labour. Third, patients may offer to do something. A fourth mode of entry is where something is offered for something else in exchange. Fifth, teaching the patient may be a way of getting the patient to work more effectively on his or her own behalf. Strauss *et al* (1985) argue that although some of patients' work is recognized by the staff as genuine, most of the 'work' undertaken by patients when they are in hospital goes unrecognized. Implicit patient work includes tasks relating to personal housekeeping, provision of information, reporting of discomforts and untoward symptoms, work associated with various tests in addition to self-control in the face of discomfort, pain and potentially humiliating medical interventions. According to Strauss *et al.*, another reason for the non-recognition of patients' work is when it is not visible to personnel. Patients may not indicate their work for a variety of reasons: because it could be defined as illegitimate, because it involves criticism of the staff, or because it is altogether too personal. My concern in this section is with the explicit work of patients on the wards.

When I started the fieldwork in the autumn of 1994 I was struck by the extent to which patients were engaged in their care compared with my own experiences of nursing only six years previously. Patients had always undertaken mundane housekeeping tasks in the hospitals in which I had worked, but what was new was their involvement in elements of their care, which, in the past, would have been carried out by nurses. I have identified three main areas where shifts in the boundary between nurses and patients had taken place: elimination products work, record-keeping and technical tasks. These are not distinct categories, however; it will become apparent that there are some areas of overlap.

Elimination products work

Much of the work undertaken by patients involved the handling of elimination products. On Treetops many patients routinely maintained their own fluid balance charts. This entailed measuring and recording fluid intake and output and, in some cases, assessing and recording the colour of their urine. Patients with renal colic filtered their urine for kidney stones. On the medical ward, people with gastric disorders weighed and recorded bowel movements and collected stool specimens.

The products of elimination assume a special place in the culture of all social groups (Douglas 1966; Loudon 1977; Lawler 1991). According to Douglas (1966) the body is an important symbol of society. Its margins symbolize the boundaries of the community and are therefore potentially polluting. There are no human societies where the acts of excretion are not subject to normative expectations of some kind. Loudon (1977, cited by Lawler 1991: 77) argues that in childhood, people learn to be positive or neutral about their own excreta and negative to that of others. As Dunlop (1986) observes, to care for another's pollution is a restatement of humility and love. Sharing dirt assumes a knowledge and friendship with a person. Nursing involves, *inter alia,* the handling of body products and the management of leaky bodies. In the course of their everyday work nurses have to transcend pollution taboos and cross sensitive social boundaries (Lawler 1991; Littlewood 1991). Ward staff at Woodlands maintained that patients preferred to handle their own dirt and thus, at one level certainly, the involvement of patients in elimination products work was oriented to minimizing their embarrassment.

> *The chaps – I don't think a lot like giving you the urine – they like to do it themselves.*
>
> (HCA)

JUNIOR SISTER: We're just needing two more FOBs [stool specimens] off her. She's got the pots because she doesn't like us doing it. She doesn't want us to do it. She did give me a sample last night but it only covered the spatula so I said 'it's not enough.' So she is aware. She doesn't like her bowels.

(Handover – Tape)

Indeed, patients could inadvertently create more work for staff by trying to carry out their own elimination products work.

JUNIOR SISTER: But she tries to do things for herself and she won't let the girls help her. She insisted on doing her bag [changing a colostomy bag] herself this morning and she didn't get it on properly and so it leaked and so she wouldn't let the girls help clean her up and so she got into a bit of a state about that. We try to help her but she won't let us.

(Handover – Tape)

At another level, however, it is also noteworthy that these were poten-tially very time-consuming activities and for nurses to have undertaken these tasks themselves would have greatly increased their burdens of work. In fact when we actually look at nurses' accounts of these shifts in the division of labour, we see that workload issues and ideologies of patient empowerment are intertwined.

> [T]hey wee in a bottle. It's marked at the bottom and unless they've got very bad eye-sight there's no reason at all why they can't measure their own urine. I mean even taking it to the sluice and emptying it out and cleaning the bottle out there's nothing to it. We show them how to do it. A lot of them are quite happy they like to do it. Then they go back and they mark it off on their charts and they feel really involved in their care. Well why shouldn't they? It's their body, it's their operation, it's their care. So I quite like it. I like this ward for that. You don't hear many buzzers going off on this ward.
>
> (Staff Nurse)

Record-keeping

Much of the elimination products work undertaken by patients entailed a record-keeping component, but patients also undertook record-keeping work of other kinds. For example, some patients kept an account of the food they had eaten. There were also various charts on which they were asked to document details of their pain – indicating the location, severity and type of pain and its relationship to other activities of daily living such as eating. As with the elimination products work, however, when we scrutinize nurses' explanations of patients' involve-ment in record-keeping, the discourse of patient participation is again woven together with a discourse of work.

> [T]hey record them (fluid balance) more accurately than we do because usually we only go round about every 4 hours [...] So the fluid charts tend to be more accurate if they do it than if we do it and it gives them something to do and it gets them involved.
>
> (Staff Nurse)

Technical tasks

The third type of work in which patients were becoming more involved was technical tasks. Firstly, patients were involved in technical work where these were new skills they would require on discharge from hospital. For example, many of the patients on the urology ward had to return home with an indwelling urethral catheter and had to know how to care for it. Secondly, those patients who had the requisite skills and/ or whose day-to-day management of chronic disorders entailed technical medical work were encouraged to use their expertise, if their condition permitted. For example, diabetic patients carried on measuring their blood sugar levels and administering their own insulin. To those unfamiliar with hospital routine, this may all sound commonsensical, but, in the past, nurses would have expected to have performed these tasks for the patient while they were in hospital and as such, these changes represent an important shift in practice.

Unlike elimination products work and record keeping, workload issues did not appear to be a dominant concern in nurses' accounts of the delegation of technical tasks to patients. Rather, patient involvement in this area of work was much more closely bound up with notions of self-management. Nevertheless, reduction in the length of hospital admissions has clearly increased the need for patients to develop technical expertise to support early discharge, and so even though workload issues did not figure prominently in nurses' talk, we cannot discount them entirely in our analysis.

At one level then, compared with my own nursing experience, the boundary between nurses and patients appeared to be changing at Woodlands. Patients were certainly more actively involved in the provision of their care than they had been when I was in clinical practice and their personal knowledge and self-management skills were clearly recognized by staff. These shifts way from the traditional passive patient role were accomplished through a combination of direct face-to-face negotiation, the provision of educational material and information leaflets, and indirectly by patients taking their cues from others on the ward. This last point clearly raises the question as to whether some of the patients fully understood what they were doing when they undertook self-care activities. Moreover, how nurses judged patients to be capable of participating in health care work was far from clear and, as such, this is an area that warrants further research.

The case of care planning

Although most of the patients seemed happy to undertake discrete tasks they were less willing to involve themselves in the planning of care. As we have seen, this was a major organizational concern and was regularly audited by senior nurses. Yet here nurses' efforts to involve patients in the caring division of labour were largely unsuccessful. The nurse–patient boundary was not a theme I had anticipated at the start of the research and, as a consequence I did not interview patients about their views of the changes that were taking place. Ethical approval had not been obtained and limitations of time and resources were also prohibitive. Thus a degree of caution needs to be exercised in seeking explanations for these findings. However, one possible reason for patients' reluctance to involve themselves in care planning may have been the threat that this posed to the traditional nurse–patient role. By undertaking discrete tasks it was possible for patients to feel that they were helping the nurses, but to assume care planning work was to erode the traditional asymmetries of expertise in the lay–professional relationship. Indeed there appears to be some support for such an interpretation in the literature. For example, Darbyshire's (1994) work on parental participation on paediatric wards suggests that parents saw their participation in the work primarily in terms of helping the nurses, and the work of Caress (1997) on renal patients indicates that even after years of self-management patients did not feel they had the requisite knowledge to be involved in decision-making about their care. Ersser (1997) has also underlined the lack of congruence in nurses' and patients' perceptions of the therapeutic effects of patient-involvement in care: nurses believed patient participation to be beneficial but patients did not. It is also noteworthy that patients' refusal to participate in care planning was not a source of tension. Given the importance of care planning as a symbol of partnerships in care one could reasonably have expected this to be the case. Arguably, however, it was easier for nurses to plan the care without the patient.

In the light of these findings, then, it is difficult to resist the conclusion that those shifts in the division of labour that had successfully taken place were as much a reflection of workload considerations and the need to plug gaps in the service, as they were any commitment to partnerships in care. Indeed recent evidence suggests that relatives on both sides of the Atlantic are also undertaking care in hospital settings because of the perceived shortage of nursing staff (Glazer 1993; Lipley 1999). In the North American context, Brannon (1994) has argued that the intensification of care brought about by the shift to primary nursing in an era of cost-containment in health service provision, led to nurses shifting tasks previously performed by auxiliaries onto patients and their families. Indeed, analysis of the processes of negotiation on the wards at Woodlands indicated that both patients and nurses subscribed to a moral division of labour that had more in keeping with that described by Parsons, than it did contemporary ideologies of caring.

Exploring the limits of change: negotiating the 'moral division of labour' between nurses and patients

Kelly and May (1982) and May and Kelly (1982) have suggested that the diverse patients who come to be typified by nurses as 'bad' are united by a common theme: their refusal to legitimate the nursing role. In this sense, then, 'bad' patients are rather like nurses' dirty work designations – they are a reflection of a particular occupational perspective and professional identity. Given the reconstruction of the nurse–patient boundary in nursing's professional discourse, the logic of Kelly and May and May and Kelly's argument would lead us to expect that patients who refused to participate in caring partnerships with nurses would be deemed problematic by staff: as they are effectively denying nurses the possibility of carrying out their work in accordance with their professional ideologies. Yet analysis of the interaction between nurses and patients in my data does not support this. On the contrary, difficulties arose when negotiation of the nurse–patient boundary threatened to undermine *traditional* role relationships. The main problems centred on issues of nurses' professional legitimacy and their control over the caring process.

Medications

Administration of medications was a particularly sensitive area. Patients who questioned their medications were a potential source of friction.

> *Patients that ask about their drugs they're always seen as trouble-makers.*

> (Student)

Rather than accepting patient enquiries about their drugs as an expression of their involvement and interest in their care (which would be in line with the new partnership models), the nurses appeared to regard such work as illegitimate. It seemed that the nurses interpreted patient's questions as implying a lack of trust in their professional competence. Patients' awareness of the sensitivity of this role boundary was evident in their interactions with nurses.

> On the drugs round one of the patients asked if she could have something for her bowels. Staff nurse said, 'We'll get you something written up.' The patient said, 'I'll tell you what suits me best if you don't mind me saying and that's glycerine suppositories.' Staff nurse said, 'We can't give you anything until the doctor writes it up.'

The patient's interactional strategy in this data extract clearly indicates that she recognizes that in making a suggestion about her medication she is moving into delicate territory, as indicated by her use of the mitigator – 'if you don't mind me saying.' Her suspicions are apparently confirmed when the nurse does not acknowledge the patient's suggestion in any way, she simply asserts the power of the doctor and the hospital rules. As I have argued, the refashioning of the nurse–patient relationship in professional nursing discourse runs against the grain of the orthodox model of lay–professional relations and yet rather than working with 'new nursing' models of partnership, it would seem that nurses' actions were oriented to the traditional asymmetries of the orthodox professional archetype. Given nurses' subordinate position in the health services division of labour, it may be the case that, at present, their professional identity is simply too fragile to accommodate ideologies of partnership in daily practice.

Technical equipment

There were also strains that related to the monitoring of equipment by patients. This was particularly the case on the surgical ward, where technology was a highly visible component of patient care. The issues here were subtly different from those associated with patients who monitored their medications. It was not that nurses felt patient involvement in technical care was illegitimate, in fact they actually encouraged patients to monitor medical equipment, but like the patients who monitored their medication, those who surveyed their technical equipment also ran the risk of implying a lack of trust in nursing staff. Moreover, the patients who engaged in over-enthusiastic monitoring and repeatedly called for nursing attention created more work for nurses, disrupted their work organization and undermined their control over work priorities.

> You'll say 'Keep your eye on your catheter. If it goes dark tell us and we'll come and alter your bladder irrigation', and then they'll sit and they're watching their bladder irrigation dripping, dripping, dripping. 'It's stopped dripping nurse.' [frustrated voice] 'I've switched it off! I don't want it to drip.' [...]'This bottle's empty!', 'My catheter's full!' and that's when I feel like saying 'Shut up!', but they're only trying to make your job easier. They're trying to help and we don't look at it like that. You sometimes feel as though they're interfering. They are interfering it's their care isn't it but we've had the odd patient or two that's not left you alone.
>
> (Staff Nurse)

On a number of occasions during the course of the fieldwork I observed patients who were perceived to be 'demanding' moved to different areas of the ward from where nursing staff would be less readily visible.

STAFF NURSE: He's a little bit [lowers voice] awkward at times. And we've moved him down [to a bed further down the ward away from the nurses' station] because his family's at you all the time. Playing with everything [technical equipment]. So we've moved him down.

(Nursing handover – Tape)

Once again, then, these findings are at odds with new models of caring, which aim to augment patient control over the caring process.

Service or servant?

A further major source of nurse–patient tension related to patients' requests for staff to undertake activities for them that the nurses believed they ought to perform for themselves. Here professional expertise, control over the work process and issues of occupational identity interacted in complex ways to produce strains. Lawler (1991) has pointed out that nurses have a very 'task-specific' approach to what they regard as situations when patients need assistance. Lawler identifies a recovery trajectory similar to the dying trajectory described by Glaser and Strauss (1968). During the recovery trajectory nurses negotiate the 'handing back' of control over the body. According to Lawler, the recovery trajectory follows a pattern and timetable that is predominantly set by the nurse rather than the patient. Variations in this pattern can cause problems. Lawler's findings appeared to be supported in this study.

Some patients could take too long to recover, leading nurses to exert pressure on them to resume their normal activities.

> *We've got a lady at the moment who likes to go to the toilet on the bedpan when she's quite able to walk – it's slow and it's a little bit painful for her to walk but if we can keep them walking we prefer to do that.*

(Staff Nurse)

STUDENT: She had a steroid injection into her knee this morning so she's on 24-hour bed-rest. So she can now use the commode legally!

(Handover – Tape)

158

Other patients tried to recover too quickly, which created concern amongst the nursing staff for their physiological well-being.

> A patient wanders out of bay one with his wash things and a towel in his hands.
> PATIENT: Sister I've just come up from coronary care. Is it OK if I have a shower?
> JUNIOR SISTER: Umm ha – umm when did you come up?
> PATIENT: Today.
> JUNIOR SISTER: When did you come in?
> PATIENT: Tuesday. I can leave it until tomorrow if you like.
> JUNIOR SISTER: If you would. I'd prefer it tomorrow. I'm on in the morning.

According to Lawler, nurses' ideas about appropriate recovery trajectories are based almost exclusively on the patient's medical condition. However, my data indicate that a further factor seems to be in play. On the whole, those patients who tried to do too much did not cause the same sorts of tension as those who were perceived to do too little. I suggest, therefore, that these findings indicate that patient recovery trajectories may also be understood in terms of nurses' expectations of the sick role. In Parson's classic model, which was based on the professional perspective, there is an expectation that the sick person *wants* to get better and should co-operate with health professionals in doing so. At Woodlands, those patients who tried to do too much were at least meeting one of these expectations, whereas those who did too little were meeting neither. Moreover, those patients who did too little undermined nurses' professional identity. A striking feature of the accounts ward staff gave of their work was the recurrence of the service analogy.

> Gill [staff nurse] came out of the ladies' bay looking harassed. I gave her an inquiring look. She beckoned me into the sluice. 'That woman in bed 2 is driving me mad,' she announced. 'Every time I go anywhere near her bed she is asking me to do something.' Gill said that this particular patient had asked her to turn the television down. 'There's no reason why she can't get up and turn the television down herself' [...] I don't come into work to run around turning the TV down. That's not what nursing's about is it? I'm not a bloody servant.' [I smiled sympathetically]

The nursing handover was a central mechanism through which nurses and support workers were able to 'stage' (Levy 1982) their negotiations with patients. This ensured that expectations of patients were consistent and constituted an important mechanism through which staff were able to consolidate their power to set the pace of 'normal' recovery and thus the nurse–patient division of labour. There are obvious resonances here with the findings of Parker *et al.* (1992), who have pointed to the ways in which nurses develop stereotypes of patients at handover. Notwithstanding these considerations, however, it is evident that participatory models of caring throw up important dilemmas in relation to patient recovery, namely, who controls it and who is ultimately accountable for the outcome? At the time of the research, control over patient recovery remained, for the most part, with nursing staff. Yet it was also clear that the consumerist climate in health care had left nurses feeling increasingly constrained in negotiating what they considered to be a legitimate allocation of work with their patients.

Of course, it would be all too easy to be critical of the nurses for this discrepancy between their theory and practice. Indeed as May and Kelly (1982) observe, much of the literature on 'problem' patients – especially that which is written for and by nurses – has a highly moral tone. The labelling of patients as a 'problem' is deemed to reflect unprofessional attitudes that need to be addressed by educational interventions. Few seem to consider that 'problem' patients are so defined because they make staff's life difficult (see also Rosenthal *et al.* 1980; Murcott 1981). Moreover, there is some evidence to suggest that when the available services are restricted there is a tendency for health care professionals to formulate patients in negative ways. For example, Stearns (1991) describes how mechanisms designed to control the costs of medical care that restricted the clinical options open to the doctor resulted in more patients being perceived as demanding as they fell outside the available alternatives. At Woodlands, a single nurse could be responsible for the care of up to seventeen patients on a given shift. I suggest, therefore, that rather than being a straightforward indicator of nurses' reluctance to change their relationships with patients, the 'problem' patient designations of nursing staff must also be understood as a reflection of the difficulties nurses faced in accommodating individual patient needs within the practical constraints of the work setting.

Conclusions

In this chapter I have extended the analytic framework employed in the analysis of nursing's occupational boundaries to examine the changing division of labour between nurses and patients. My data suggest that patients were becoming increasingly involved in the caring division of labour in the study site and in many areas their knowledge and skills were being recognized. These changes are clearly an important move away from the passivity of the traditional patient role, but we should be cautious about proclaiming a radical shift in the caring relationship. Drawing on the work of Hughes, I have suggested that although nurses and patients appeared to have accommodated shifts in the allocation of tasks, changes to their role-relationship were more problematic. Moreover, what shifts in the caring division of labour that had successfully taken place, appeared to reflect the need to plug gaps in the service as much as they did contemporary ideologies of lay–professional partnerships. Changes to the caring division of labour were also limited by the differential knowledge of nurses and patients, the practical constraints of caring on hospital wards, and the perceptions of nurses and patients of their respective roles.

9

CONCLUSIONS

There are so many recent initiatives that are bringing pressure
to bear on nurses. When I sit and think about it I think about
the Hillsborough disaster and people being shoved up against
the fence and I feel a bit like that about what's happening to
nursing. [...] I know it's a little bit of a cruel sort of an analogy
but I do feel a bit like that about it.

(Nurse Manager)

I began this book with the juxtaposition of two quotations that reflected
the tension between professional and management versions of nursing,
and I have examined the ways in which, at a particular point in time and
in a particular context, these discourses interacted to fashion the shape
of nursing work in daily practice. Throughout this text I have employed
a non-essentialist conceptualization of nursing work. I have argued that
nursing jurisdiction is done, and that the boundaries of nursing work are
produced through the locally situated actions and interactions in which
nurses engage in the course of their daily practice. What is also clear,
however, is that nursing jurisdiction is not accomplished in circumstances of nurses' own choosing. The nurse manager's words that open
this concluding chapter are a powerful – albeit controversial – expression of the constraints experienced by staff in the course of their
everyday work.

In this final chapter I attempt a synthesis of the study's findings and
evaluate the consequences of nurses' boundary management for their
occupational jurisdiction. Whereas the empirical chapters have concentrated on interactional processes, here the focus shifts to 'shape' and
'shapers'. I end with an examination of developments since this study
was undertaken, and consider their possible implications for the
changing shape of nursing practice.

Doing nursing at Woodlands Hospital

The routine construction of nursing boundaries at Woodlands was influenced by a range of factors. Nurses had to accomplish their work against a backdrop of economic stringency. Care had to be provided with a mixture of nurses, students in training and support workers, and the skill and grade mix of staff on the wards had important implications for the division of labour that was possible, and hence, the shape of nursing work. Ward nurses were responsible for up to seventeen patients, which made it difficult to provide individualized care and establish satisfactory relationships with them. Meeting the 'named nurse' standard in any meaningful sense was almost impossible, and yet the need for 'ceremonial compliance' (Heimer 1998) with this quality standard placed an additional demand on nurses' time and energy. In fact the pressures of work on staff were such that even patients and their relatives[1] were being co-opted into the division of labour in order to plug gaps in the service.

A further constraint nurses faced was the new consumerist culture in health care. It entered into their negotiations with patients and was an important source of tension. The recurrence of the service metaphor in nurses' accounts highlighted their difficulties in negotiating patient recovery and encouraging independence. Nurses also believed that consumerism had increased public expectations of the service. While they were sympathetic to many of their demands, they had insufficient resources to meet them, which was demoralizing.

> *I think it's with the 'Patient's Charter'. Patients demand more which is quite fair enough but the provisions aren't there to meet their demands so it's the nurses that get it in the neck because they're not meeting the demands but there's no provision's been made to meet those demands. So you come away feeling inadequate and picked on. It sounds really pathetic but picked on. I don't know when management come and you tell them there's no staff but you have to just carry on. So you really work yourself hard and you get no recognition for that. It's just the whole collective you know and it's coming to that and it's like a boil festering and it's coming to a head at the moment and it's going to erupt.*
>
> (Staff Nurse)

Given the daily reality of nursing work, it is hardly surprising that the expansion of the support-worker boundary was accomplished with relative ease at ward level, even if this was in tension with the professional vision. Indeed the pressures of work on the wards had already resulted in the informal blurring of this interface prior to the introduction of the HCA role. At least with its formalization, the HCAs had a more thorough educational preparation for the work they were expected to undertake and had been equipped with a vocabulary of 'risk' with which to resist the allocation of work for which they felt inadequately prepared.

Paperwork was a further restriction on the shape of nurses' work because it was so time consuming. Management emphasis on quality assurance, coupled with the fear of litigation, meant that considerable effort went into what I have described as the paper construction of nursing care. Here we saw how the discourses of professionalism and managerialism intersected in powerful ways to fashion the content of nurses' work. The nursing care plan became an important mechanism through which the 'quality' of nursing was monitored in the organization and ceremonial compliance with standards realized. Yet, because care plans are founded on a rather different version of nursing work from the real life of hospital wards, they had little practical value for nurses and their satisfactory completion was an additional demand on their time, which further removed them from sustained patient contact.

Another constraint on nurses' actions was their relative power in the organization. Medical dominance was evident in the ways in which nurses accomplished jurisdiction on the wards and also in terms of the composition of the principal decision-making arenas at Woodlands. As we saw in Chapter 7, although at ward level nurses were prepared to negotiate the division of labour with individual doctors and wielded considerable influence over treatment decisions, this took place against the backdrop of the overall hegemony of the institution of medicine. For example, nurses' informal boundary-blurring work can be understood, in part, as a reflection of the strains that arose out of the disjuncture between the flow of work and the formal authority structure. Quite simply it was easier for nurses to undertake the work themselves than it was to try and negotiate from a subordinate position with over-burdened doctors who had different priorities and perspectives.

We have also seen how nurses' power was constrained in the key policy-making arenas at Woodlands. The Director of Nursing was the lone nursing voice on the Hospital Management Board – which was numerically dominated by doctors as directors of the clinical management teams, all but one of whom were men. Traynor (1999) has highlighted the ways in which the views of nurses are marginalized by management discourse. The nurse managers at Woodlands expressed the opinion that it was extremely difficult for them to get nursing issues discussed at Trust management meetings. The Director of Nursing described how she often had to resort to tacking nursing concerns onto other items on the agenda, which were afforded higher priority – such as risk management. Furthermore, changes to the clinical management team structure initiated by the Chief Executive looked likely further to mute the nursing voice. Nurses' powerlessness in these key arenas at Woodlands clearly had important implications for ward level staff because it was here that decisions, which were highly consequential for the environment in which they functioned, were made.

Organizational turbulence has been a recurring theme in this book. At one level, this turbulence reflects the centrality of the patient, which as Strauss *et al.* (1985) point out, makes medical work fundamentally non-rationalizable. At another level, hospitals are complex, internally segmented organizations and patient care has to be provided around the clock, throughout the year, by different care providers and co-ordinated with numerous internal and external timetables which are often in conflict (Zerubavel 1979; Wolf 1988). I have argued that comprehending this context is vital to understanding why nurses make their work boundaries in the shape that they do, but it is a feature of the daily reality of hospital nursing that has hitherto been ignored by policy makers and nursing leaders in the debates over the nursing role.

Owing to their working environment, hospitals need a point of flexibility in the system in order to function and there is a sense in which a 'usefulness' culture underpins hospital life. Yet the imperative to be 'flexible' or 'useful' is not shared equally by all hospital workers. It is nurses who are expected to be the malleable workers in the system and this constrains the shape of their jurisdiction in important ways. Unlike the periodic contact of most other categories of hospital worker, nurses are present with the patient continuously. Study after study has shown that nurses do not worry themselves too deeply about demarcation issues (Ball and Goldstone 1987; Beardshaw and Robinson 1990; Davies 1995). Indeed, it is likely that most would consider it 'unprofessional' to do so. Rather, nurses undertake whatever is necessary in order to provide the care for their patients. There is evidence to suggest, however, that nurses' willingness to blur the boundaries of their formal jurisdiction is subject to abuse by work overload (Corley and Mausksch 1988; Hart 1989). In the policy-making arena, there seems to be an assumption that nursing work is infinitely elastic and that, as the largest occupational group, the nursing work force represents an endlessly absorbent sponge ready to soak-up every additional duty. At Woodlands certainly, flexibility was an institutionalized expectation of the nursing role.

For example, in Chapter 7 I argued that although individual nurse practitioner posts at Woodlands had been resourced through funds that had been made available through the junior doctors' hours initiative, there was no money to support ward-based staff in the development of their jurisdiction. The expectation was that nurses would just absorb these new activities into their existing work. Owing to the turbulence of the work environment, undertaking medically-derived tasks had a certain organizational logic – it was often easier for nurses to carry out some activities than to expend energy trying to get the doctor to come to the ward – and it definitely had benefits for patient care. This helps to account for the ease with which shifts in the nursing–medical interface were made at ward-level, despite objections raised elsewhere in the profession. Equally, however, I have argued that because of the need to work with a variable mix of staff and manage multiple patient assign-ments in response to the complex temporal structures of the hospital, nurses found it hard to involve themselves in any sustained patient contact work. Indeed, many were loathe to engage in prolonged care activities lest their skills were needed elsewhere. Not only did this make it difficult for them to establish the sorts of inter-personal relationships with patients, which they regarded as a central reward of the job, it also undermined their sense of professional competence because of the obstacles the work organization presented for getting 'to know the patient'. At the same time, however, the unpredictability of patients also meant that it was utterly impractical for nurses to have attempted to create more time for hands-on care by divesting themselves of all mundane work activities.

Taken together, then, these inter-related constraints constituted the structural context in which nurses at Woodlands managed their work boundaries and, as we have seen, this had important implications for the shape of nursing's workplace jurisdiction. It encouraged the blurring of the nurse–support worker boundary and the nursing–medical interface despite the problems this posed for nurses' occupational identities. Nurses at all levels of the organization were realistic as to how far the ideals of the profession were achievable in practice, and had accommo-dated themselves to a mode of work organization that might best be described as pragmatic professionalism. Nevertheless, ward-based staff faced real difficulties in negotiating a satisfactory work role. For example, although some nurses were equivocal about the level of inti-macy implied by certain versions of the nurse–patient relationship, spending time with their patients was regarded as an important reward of the job that was always frustratingly out of their reach. We also saw the difficulties nurses experienced in attempting to implement a 'profes-sional' model of autonomous practice in the hospital context and the interpersonal strains that this created on both wards relating to 'knowing the patient', control over the work and an equitable division of labour.

Additionally, the professional ideal of the autonomous practitioner presented problems for staff working within a bureaucratic organization.

This study was undertaken at a particular point in time and in a particular context. Almost a decade has passed since the introduction of Project 2000 and the 1990 NHS and Community Care Act, and much has happened in the intervening period. A new political party has taken office and once again the health service is undergoing reform. The internal market has been abolished and is being replaced by a 'third way' hybrid, which lies somewhere between a command and control structure based on hierarchies on the one hand, and markets and competition on the other (Hunter 1998). The political rhetoric has shifted from one framed predominantly in terms of notions of cost, competition, consumerism and efficiency, to a vocabulary that embraces ideals of partnership, quality and the incorporation of user views into service planning. The Health Service is poised to enjoy a period of 'sustained investment' (DH 2000a) and central to this will be the expansion of the NHS workforce. Project 2000 is being evaluated and the future of nurse education considered. The Department of Health has just published its strategy for nursing – *Making a Difference* (DH 1999c) – which has been warmly received in the nursing press. Nurses have recently enjoyed the largest pay rise in 10 years (DH 1999a) and there is the promise of a new career structure that includes 'consultant nurses', 'modern matrons' and an 'enhanced role' for nurses (DH 2000a). There has been much talk of making the NHS a more family-friendly workplace (DH 1999b). After an intensive recruitment campaign, applications to nurse training programmes are again on the increase. The mood is altogether more buoyant than the one that provided the backdrop to this study, but will any of this affect nurses' ability to negotiate a satisfactory occupational role? In the final section of the book I take a look at recent developments in the UK health care scene and consider their implications for the future shape of nursing work.

The future shape of nursing work?

The changing division of labour in the provision of health services remains high on the current policy agenda and is unlikely to go away as health care systems across the developed world are reformed and restructured in order to respond to the demands of the twenty-first century. The issue of work roles and responsibilities recurs regularly in discussions of cost-effectiveness, quality, national and international professional and inter-professional regulation. And despite being given a softer focus in New Labour rhetoric, the discourse of managerialism continues to be a powerful force in shaping these debates.

Junior doctors' hours remain a concern. Acknowledging that the *New Deal* (NHSME 1991) had only been partially successful, the Government and British Medical Association recently announced a new agreement that, in line with the European Union working time directive, will cut the maximum hours junior doctors work to 48 per week over a 13-year period. Over the next three years efforts will be made to reduce all junior doctors' hours to no more than 56 hours per week (DTI 1999). It is highly likely that further ways of managing the workload in hospital settings will have to be considered and once again nursing has entered into the equation (DH 1999c).

Although some concerns have been raised in the letters pages of the nursing press, the nursing response to the implications of the new initiative on junior medical staff hours has, on the whole, been curiously muted. Indeed, the furore over nurses becoming 'mini' doctors, which characterized the political climate of the early 1990s, appears to have been replaced by a degree of resignation that the medical–nursing boundary has shifted – in some areas permanently.

> As particular tasks have become commonplace, e.g. intravenous drug administration and cannulation, they have been subsumed into nursing, midwifery and health visiting in many areas and form, following relevant preparation, the expected skills base of registered practitioners.
>
> (UKCC 1999a: 1)

Reporting for *The Nursing Times* on the findings of a UKCC study of the implementation of *The Scope of Professional Practice*, which revealed that 33 per cent of the nurses it surveyed were unaware of its existence, Coombes (2000) writes:

> Sadly, the report suggests many nurses are missing out on exciting career opportunities because of an inability to act on the scope of professional practice.
>
> (Coombes 2000: 4)

And a further recent article accused the government of 'hijacking [...] good practice developed by health professionals and their managers over the last decade, presenting them as innovations spawned by the government' (Mahony 2000: 10).

To a considerable extent then, it would seem that the debates appear to be moving away from the question as to whether nurses should be undertaking medically-derived work, to centre on the issue of how the plethora of posts and titles that have evolved in the wake of the junior doctors' hours initiative and the *Scope of Professional Practice* (UKCC 1992) should be regulated and standards safeguarded. The UKCC is considering a new level of registration for those nurses working 'at a higher level of practice' (UKCC 1999a; UKCC 1999b) and the consultative documents it has issued indicate a degree of acceptance of the inevitability of evolving boundaries across all areas of nursing work and a rejection of a simplistic task-based skills hierarchy. For example, the descriptor of the higher level of practice is to identify *how* practitioners work at this level rather than simply concentrating on what they do. The exercise has been couched primarily in terms of the need to safeguard standards and protect the public, yet it may also be read as an important political move that attempts to retain professional control over nursing jurisdiction. The lack of standardization in the roles of nurses working 'at a higher level of practice' makes it extremely difficult for them to transfer their skills to other organizations. Given current policy trends, however, the UKCC faces a formidable task.

The concept of flexible working seems to have become something of an orthodoxy in health policy circles, reflecting the ascendancy of post-Fordist management ideologies in both manufacturing and service industries. Although these new forms of work organization – just in time, total quality management, business process re-engineering and human resource management – differ in certain key respects, there is a common link. That is, they have allowed, or provided a rationale for, wide-ranging changes in the way work is organized, especially breaking down lines of demarcation (Strangleman and Roberts 1999). In the NHS under new public management, changes in the division of labour have been justified in the interests of both efficiency and quality and recent policy developments indicate a strong continuation of this overall trend. The notion of flexible working is woven throughout the policy papers of the four government health departments (DH 1998; Scottish Office and Department of Health 1997; Welsh Office and NHS Cymru Wales 1998; DHSS Northern Ireland 1998), it is central to the *NHS Plan* (DH 2000a) and Chapter 10 of *Making a Difference* makes it clear that 'there is no place for rigid demarcation of role boundaries in a modern service' (DH 1999c: 70). The recent publication of the consultative document *A Health Service of all the Talents* (DH 2000b) by the Department of Health in England takes these overall trends a step further, sign-posting a future of further blurred professional boundaries, new types of health care worker and an educational system which would facilitate 'flexible careers', that is, movement between one occupation and another. The idea of a single regulating body for all health professionals has been mooted in a number of arenas. So what are the implications of these so-called 'new ways of working' for nurses?

At one level, proponents of 'new nursing' would certainly be heart-ened by the patient-centred vignettes of nursing practice cited in *Making a Difference* (DH 1999c), *The NHS Plan* (DH 2000a) and *A Health Service of all the Talents* (DH 2000b) as exemplars of the government's vision for 'joined-up' health provision. Moreover, coupled with the current emphasis on 'user-involvement' these trends would appear to indicate that policy makers have heeded the call made by a number of authors in recent years of the need for a new model of professionalism in health care (see, for example, Stacey 1992; Witz 1994; Davies 1995) that is based on engagement and partnership rather than the detachment and inequalities of the orthodox paradigm, and that recognizes the contribution of other members of the multidisciplinary team. Arguably, nurses have long embraced many of these ideals, but the context in which they work has made it extremely difficult for them to put this into practice. Will the 'New NHS' provide a context in which nurses are able to proactively develop their roles around patients' needs and develop partnerships in care or will the other forces in play leave them feeling that important elements of their work have dropped through the hole in the middle?

A key development likely to impact upon the contours of nursing work in the UK is the introduction of clinical governance. Here, inter-estingly, the overall direction of policy appears to be moving in the direction of (Fordist) standardization. One of the main recommenda-tions of the consultation document *A First Class Service: Quality in the New NHS* (DH 1998d) is 'a framework through which local organiza-tions are accountable for continuously improving the quality of their services and safeguarding high standards of care by creating an environ-ment in which excellence in clinical care will flourish' (p. 33). For the first time the government will systematically appraise interventions before they are introduced into the NHS and national service frame-works will set standards for a range of client groups. Health service provision will be 'evidence-based' although the precise characteristics of the 'evidence' on which services will be founded is uncertain (Closs and Cheater 1999; McKenna *et al.* 2000). McKenna *et al.* (2000) outline a number of formulations of evidence-based practice that range from narrow definitions focused entirely on research 'evidence' (Appleby *et al.* 1995) to broader conceptualizations that embrace the views of clients (McKibbon and Walker 1994).

These developments have been welcomed by some as an important shift in emphasis from the previous administration where cost saving measures were rewarded and no satisfactory attempt was made to measure the quality of care provided (Black 1998). Others, however, have pointed out that the apparently collaborative tone of *A First Class Service* has a strong element of compulsion that might potentially threaten the future of professional self-regulation. Described by one Health Authority Chief Executive as 'the biggest assault on doctors since the creation of the NHS' (NHS Confederation 2000), clinical governance may be seen as a further extension of the state's efforts to tighten administrative and cultural control over health professionals. It is far from clear, for example, to what extent the climate of the 'New NHS' will permit the exercise of clinical judgement in mediating national standards in order to meet the needs of individuals. Moreover, although much of the attention has thus far centred on treatment interventions, both *A Health Service of all the Talents* (DH 2000b) and *The NHS Plan* (DH 2000a) make it clear that the clinical governance framework extends to the organization of health services. If the proposals of *A Health Service of all the Talents* come to fruition, in the future we may see an era of 'evidence-based' service provision led by 'National Workforce Development Boards' (DH 2000b) and supported by 'Care Group Development Boards' in which national standards are developed that specify the preferred division of roles and responsibilities for particular client groups. The potential implications of these proposals for the health services division of labour are indeed profound. Furthermore, although in the short term the health service professions may continue to enjoy self-regulation, the clinical governance framework has emerged as a powerful parallel force. Given the potential of the clinical governance framework to encroach upon their professional autonomy, the response of the health care professions has been curiously muted. It may well be, that the less adversarial tone of the New Labour government (Webb 1999) and its patient-centred rhetoric has made it possible for them to drive forward policies that the Conservative government struggled to promote despite clear continuities in their overall thrust.

So what are the likely implications of clinical governance for nursing? Although the government has committed itself to reducing unnecessary bureaucracy in the health service, there is a danger that clinical governance will herald yet more systems of audit that will compound the burgeoning volume of paperwork with which front-line staff must contend. There is now a pressing need, as Power (1999) observes, for an evaluation of the effects of the audit process on the service.

A further important challenge nurses face is the inherent tension between the sorts of standardization likely to be driven by the clinical governance agenda and their 'professional' commitment to individual-ized care. Despite the optimistic formulations of evidence-based nursing emerging in the literature (see, for example Closs and Cheater 1999; McKenna *et al*. 2000) it remains unclear as to how far nurses will feel able to assert their professional expertise in the face of contrary 'evidence' in the real world of practice. *The NHS Plan* makes much of public trust in the health professions:

> Ours is a vision of a renewed public service ethos, a system that values the dedication of staff and believes that trust is the glue that binds the NHS together.
>
> (DH 2000a: 17)

But consumerism ushered in a climate of defensiveness into the NHS and the recent vilification of the health professions in the wake of a number of high profile medical negligence cases has done much to erode the traditional public service ethos that Ministers now hanker after. Will the 'New NHS' be a place where nurses are able to develop an approach to clinical decision-making 'which links the use of current best evidence, practitioners' clinical expertise and patients' (and where appropriate, their carers') preferences' (Closs and Cheater 1999: 11) or will it result in the form of professionalism described by Hoggett (1996), in which nurses become skilled in the arts of impression management and 'performing to target, even though this may run counter to the need to do the right job' (Hoggett 1996: 24, cited by Webb 1999: 756).

One key element in the clinical governance agenda in this respect is the government's claim that service users are to be involved in the definition of 'quality'. Critics of 'new nursing' have underlined the lack of evidence that patients actually want the kind of nursing care its proponents uphold as the ideal. Yet while the assumption that patients actually want close inter-personal relationships with nurses may be empirically moot, recent work has suggested that, at the very least, the general public have a strong requirement that they should be treated as individuals (Baker and Lyne 1996; Ersser 1997). It could be here that nurses have powerful allies in underlining the value of their contribution. The new guidelines make it clear that Trust managers will be held to account if satisfactory standards are not attained, and in a recent case in Eastbourne where nursing short-ages were highlighted as a contributory factor in the death of a patient, the Trust Executive and Chairman lost their jobs (Carlin and Mahony 1999; Lambert 1999). California has recently become the first US state to impose minimum skill-mix ratios on hospitals (*Nursing Times* 1999) and it is perhaps possible that standards of this kind may be written into national service frameworks in the UK in the future.

However appealing this might be, it is far from clear whether the taxpaying public is prepared to pay for the kinds of service being assembled in contemporary health policy as the ideal. The rhetoric may have shifted away from that which characterized the early years of the managerialist era, but New Labour's continued emphasis on partnership and user involvement is equally likely to raise the public's expectations of the service. Much of the future of the 'New NHS' may be open to speculation, but one thing that is certain is that, despite the recent announcement of a programme of investment, economic stringency will continue to be an important shaper of services. Recent policy documents have a decidedly consumerist tone – for example that every patient will have a bedside TV and telephone by 2004 (DH 2000a) – and if public expectations are not matched by adequate resources then nurses will be exposed to the full force of unmet service-user demands and this will have important implications for morale and staff retention. Commenting on the public service class as a whole Webb (1999) observes:

> Each strategy to enhance responsiveness to users requires a greater degree of flexibility of labour, including greater variability of working hours, greater flexibility over tasks and higher levels of competence in routine service relationships. In the context of declining budgets, the implication is intensification of work for most and greater emotional demands on frontline staff, as they negotiate with users over expectations of service, which in practice entail 'more and more rationing' (Ian Johns, Social Services Director, Welsh City Council).
>
> (Webb 1999: 759)

It is also the case that the professional ideal of an all-qualified work force is likely to remain just that. In *Making a Difference* (DH 1999c) the government outlines its vision for the future of nurse education and training. It proposes more flexible pathways into and within nursing and midwifery education with 'stepping on' and 'stepping off' points. Health care assistants with the appropriate level of vocational qualifications will be allowed to fast-track nurse training, and nursing students will be able to interrupt their training armed with credits that allow them to work as a support worker in the NHS if they wish, and then return to complete their education at a later date. These themes are also echoed in *Fitness for Practice*, the report of the UKCC Commission for Nursing and Midwifery Education chaired by Sir Leonard Peach (UKCC 1999c).

The aim is that such a model will support the NHS in meeting its recruitment needs and reduce drop-out rates from nurse training.

All this signals a future in which nursing services will have to be provided with a far more complex configuration of staff with diverse skills and educational backgrounds. The extent of nursing's involvement in the preparation and regulation of support staff is, as yet, uncertain. *Making a Difference* (DH 1999c) refers to the development of local networks of vocational training centres in order to support its future vision of education and training and, as such, these developments have the potential to make significant inroads into professional self-regulation. They also raise important issues about the caring division of labour. If nurses are to realize their aspirations for patient-centred care then there is a pressing need to address the challenges this poses for the organization of nursing work. For many years, the attitude of the nursing leadership to support workers has been one of sustained ambivalence. To a considerable extent, the professional version of nursing practice has been built on the assumption of an all-qualified work force that is now unsustainable if, indeed, it ever was. With the issue of support worker regulation a priority issue for policy makers it may well be that these current developments are sufficiently radical to kick-start an informed debate about the nature of the relationship between nurses and support staff in which nursing will be able to free itself from narrow professional concerns to explore the implications of managing this interface for patient care. There is some evidence to suggest that developments of this kind are taking place in North America where the idea of 'practice partnerships' is taking root (Manthey 1989). The idea is based on the primary nursing model. It entails a nurse and support worker paired together caring for a group of patients on a given shift, and the allocation of work is determined by the nurse with the support worker carrying out activities for which she is judged to be competent with particular patients. Consideration of how the nurse–support worker boundary can best be managed in practice might be one way in which the tensions between professional and service versions of the role can begin to be reconciled, even if, in the process, this might involve asking searching questions about what it means to be a nurse.

Throughout this book I have argued that nursing jurisdiction is a practical accomplishment and that, to a considerable extent, its form is shaped by the arenas in which it is 'done'. We saw, for example, that at Woodlands the jurisdictional claims made by nurse managers were quite different from the ways in which ward staff routinely produced the boundaries of nursing practice. Perhaps the most profound manifestation of the situated character of nursing jurisdiction, however, is what is normally referred to as the theory–practice gap. As Melia (1987) has observed, the main base for those who subscribe to a professional view of nursing has tended to be in the educational sector among people who have little responsibility for day-to-day service provision. Although this situation may now be changing – for example, we saw that nurse managers at Woodlands espoused a version of nursing that embraced many features of the professional vision – the tension between the version of nursing work promulgated in the lecture theatre and the reality of nursing work remains a continuing problem. Having formulated the 'essence' of nursing in terms of an close inter-personal therapeutic relationship with patients in order to establish epistemological demarcation from medicine, much contemporary nursing scholarship appears to be directed at the establishment of a boundary between nursing theory and the social science disciplines on which it has so heavily drawn. A corollary of this is that certain elements of academic nursing are in danger of becoming even further removed from the daily reality of nursing practice. For example, Barker *et al.* (1995) have argued that Watson's theory of caring (1985) 'is couched in such obfuscatory, "new age" language that the concept of caring becomes a one-sided, emotional self-indulgence which has no place in human interaction and the helping relationship' (cited by Morrison and Cowley 1999: 25). Arguably, the same criticism could be levelled at others writing in this vein (see, for example, Parse 1981; Newman 1986).

Although the place of nurses and midwives in higher education looks safe for the foreseeable future, the period following the introduction of Project 2000 has witnessed a resurgence of the kinds of gendered anti-intellectualism (Allen 1997b; see, for example, Lawson 1996; Horton 1997) which have been so much a part of nursing's occupational development. Recent calls to 'bring back matron', indicate that the pressures for a return to nurse training (as opposed to education) are strong. Both *Making a Difference* (DH 1999c) and *Fitness for Practice* (UKCC 1999c) pay considerable attention to the relationship between the education and service sectors and emphasize the importance of ensuring newly qualified nurses have adequate practical skills. In *Making a Difference*, the government insists that the system of nurse training should be much more responsive to the needs of the NHS, and while continuing to emphasize the importance of strengthening professional self-regulation, it also envisages a future in which the Department of Health will take far more direct responsibility for the shape and direction of nurse and midwifery education. *Fitness for Practice* (UKCC 1999c) takes a slightly different line. It draws attention to the inherent tension between a generic education, which prepares the student to be adaptable, and training in particular skills, which enable them to function immediately on registration. It argues that, given that health care is forever changing, it is unreasonable to expect that fitness for purpose – other than in the broadest sense – should be a function of pre-registration education. It advocates the identification of competency-based learning outcomes for nurse training to be agreed by the NHS and higher education institutes. What is interesting about both these documents, however, is that they formulate the problematic relationship between service and education sectors in terms of the *practical* skills of nurses. Both highlight the need for lecturers in nursing to retain clinical credibility and advocate the further development and expansion of the lecturer-practitioner role. Yet none of this goes any way towards addressing the fundamental tensions between the professional version of nursing espoused in the lecture theatre and the reality of the work environment with which we have been concerned here.

It is sometimes suggested that the tensions of the theory–practice gap are healthy and function to ensure practitioners strive for professional ideals when there is a strain towards compromise in the work setting (see, for example, James 1992a). Yet this places the onus for resolving these strains on the individual practitioner. It is debateable as to whether nurses are adequately prepared for this, and the continuing problem of retention and returnees to practice indicates that the human costs may be unacceptably high. As Becker (1970) has argued, the symbol of profession is useful in so much as it helps people to organize their lives and embodies conceptions of what is good and worthwhile, but when that symbol becomes too divorced from the reality it becomes pathological. Not only does this make it difficult for nurses to negotiate in the key policy arenas, it also creates problems for nurses' professional identities when their conceptualization of their work is at odds with their daily practice. Thus, whilst the move to enhance the academic basis of nursing practice is to be strongly supported, there is also a need for nurse education to more faithfully reflect the reality of service provision (Allen 1997b).

To call for a close coupling of the service and education sectors is not, however, to endorse the current strain towards a return to service-led training. Nurse education of an appropriate kind is vital if practitioners are to function in a rapidly changing health service and to manage the boundaries of their work in the interests of patients. Critics of Project 2000 have raised the question as to whether recent efforts to augment the academic basis of nursing practice has moved nurses further away from patient care (Horton 1997). Given current health service trends, however, far from eroding their traditional caring ethos, the education of nurses is essential to its survival (Allen 1997b). Nevertheless, it is also the case that professional discourses have formulated nursing jurisdiction around nurse–patient relationships and have promulgated models of care that bear little resemblance to many of the contexts in which nurses work.[2] Furthermore, in so doing they have missed out a great deal of the work that nurses actually do.

The nurse–patient relationship is clearly an important element of the nursing function but it does not figure prominently in the daily reality of all nurses' work. This is not because practising nurses are not doing nursing properly, but because nursing roles are far more diverse than the 'new nursing' ideologies allow. Nurse managers and charge nurses have little direct contact with patients and yet make a vital contribution to the caring environment. Moreover, developments in some areas of the service such as decreased length of in-patient stay, the increased use of day surgery and telemedicine, also suggest that a key nursing skill is not to establish close interpersonal relationships with patients, but to engage with service users within a tightly circumscribed time-frame in order to accomplish the purposes at hand. Lyne (1998) has suggested that one way of reconceptualizing the nursing function is to consider, not what individual nurses do, but what is achieved by the nursing work force as a whole. She suggests that the nursing contribution to health care may be considered as analogous to the matrix of connective tissue.

> The connective tissue matrix supports, sustains and co-ordinates the work of specialized cells which carry out the function of the tissue. *In older histology textbooks this matrix is depicted as white space with no discernible structure, but modern texts show that it is far from an amorphous substance – it is highly structured and organized.*
>
> (Lyne 1998: 75, my emphasis)

In this book I have examined specific nursing boundaries and have considered the implications of nurses' boundary management for the content of their work. There is a sense, however, in which all nursing work is fundamentally about boundary management of some kind: nurses work at the boundary between nature and culture, at the boundary between life and death, at the boundary between individual need and organizational constraint, they deal with leaky bodies and leaky minds. They manage interagency and inter-organizational boundaries, mediate professional boundaries, negotiate with family carers and work at the boundary between self-care and other-care. This entails the combination of high levels of technical, management and interpersonal skills. Most

177

importantly, it also involves working *flexibly*. This flexibility is of two kinds: first, at the level of the individual there is the need for flexibility within a given role at a particular point in time and, second, at the level of the occupation there is a need for flexibility in terms of the evolution of nursing roles in response to the changing needs of the service.

What is so intriguing about recent developments in the health services division of labour is the extent to which flexible working is being presented as somehow new. *Making a Difference* (DH 1999c) refers to its vision of nurses' crossing professional boundaries as 'new ways of working', but, nurses are the ultimate flexible workers – both historically and in day-to-day practice – yet this has never been recompensed. On the contrary, nurses have been subject to increased dilution on the grounds that they are not efficiently deploying their skills. For example, a study published in 1996 by the Health Services Management Unit at Manchester University caused some disquiet amongst nurses when, in addressing the question, 'if we were designing the workforce today for tomorrow's health service, what would it look like?', it suggested the development of a 'generic worker' role in the health services (HSMU 1996). Citing evidence of the amount of time nurses spend on direct patient care and implying that time spent doing other kinds of work is inappropriate, the report belies a profound misunderstanding of the nature of nursing work. What this illustrates, however, is that nursing has yet to find an adequate language with which to articulate its function and thus elements of it remain invisible to those outside of the occupation or they get defined in a residual way. Take the following for example:

> [Nurses'] place in the division of labour is essentially that of doing in a responsible way whatever necessary things are in danger of not being done at all.
>
> (Hughes 1984: 308)

> We are reminded of a sheet of rolled-out dough from which the housewife has cut many cookies, which, on an aluminium sheet, are baking in the oven. What is left on the kitchen table is a network of dough which still suggests the entire original scope and area of the previously solid surface. Somehow, nursing is reminiscent of the pattern which remains after the cookies have been cut!
>
> (Mauskch 1966: 124)

To a considerable extent, the difficulties that nurses have had in communicating the work that they do, appear to arise from the fact that nursing is women's work and that the multiplicity of tasks that comprise nursing work bear similarities to domestic labour. As Gamarnikow (1978) has observed, nursing's occupational niche had its origins in the sexual division of labour in the Victorian household and, at the root of their 'professional predicament', is the challenge of developing an intellectual basis for this work (Davies 1995).

The current climate indicates that it may be possible to formulate the nursing contribution in more positive terms. There is a growing recognition that a certain level of chaos is inevitable in the health care sector (Klein 1997; cited by Lyne 1998) and that boundary management is a vital, but overlooked skill required in the successful functioning of such complex systems. Drawing on the work of Schön (1971), Hunter (1990) has pointed to the need for 'network negotiators' in modern health care settings and underlines their value in 'making [things] happen' (Harvey-Jones 1989). He argues that network managers are required who can combine highly competent technical skills with a keen sensitivity to interpersonal and group relationships. Hunter argues that '[i]nterface management *ought* to be regarded as the ultimate challenge to aspiring managers and a pinnacle of managerial achievement' (Hunter 1990: 14, emphasis in original), but currently lacks a sound theoretical and empirical research base. According to Hunter, '[t]here is much good practice in evidence. But we [...] are not very good at reflecting upon it, documenting it and drawing out the lessons of policy and practice' (Hunter 1990: 12–13). Hunter addresses his observations to a management audience, yet arguably much could be learnt from nursing. It is, perhaps, significant that Hunter refers to the concept of 'negotiated order' to express this vital reticulist (Friend, *et al.* 1974, cited by Hunter 1990) role.

To advocate a broader formulation of nursing work is not to diminish the importance of the nurse–patient relationship nor is it to suggest that nurse education should be exclusively service-led. Rather, it is to focus on the range of activities in which nurses routinely engage, the skills they deploy and the value of what they do. Central to this is flexibility. Attempts to fix the nursing role too rigidly are doomed to fail; the content of nursing practice, as the title of this book implies, is forever changing, both historically and in daily practice, and will continue to do so. This is its strength. However, if nurses are to shape and reshape their bundle of work activities in order to maximize the benefits for patients, then the challenge for the occupation is to establish empirical evidence of the nursing contribution and a vocabulary through which this can be communicated and incorporated into the educational process.

NOTES

INTRODUCTION

1 Although the term 'support worker' could legitimately be applied to a broad range of staff whose work supports nursing, I employ the term in a more limited sense to refer to auxiliaries and HCAs only.

2 In the original study I analysed the boundary between nurses and patients together with the boundary between nurses and family members and friends, limitations of space do not permit the inclusion of all this material. For further information on this work see Allen (1996, 2000)

1 PROFESSIONALISM AND MANAGERIALISM

1 At this time Eric Caines was the Personnel Director of the NHS.

2 The EN/RN distinction has parallels with the LPN/RN distinction in the US.

3 The UKCC (United Kingdom Council for Nursing, Midwifery and Health Visiting) is a statutory body responsible for the establishment of standards for training and professional conduct and the protection of the public from unsafe practice. It is charged with the responsibility for maintaining a single register of all practitioners and determining the conditions of entry. It is supported by four national boards of the four countries of the UK: England, Wales, Scotland and Northern Ireland who have responsibility for implementing UKCC policies and rules.

4 Nurses were certainly not the only group to be affected by dilution. A re-profiling exercise in the diagnostic imaging unit at Bradford Hospitals Trust led to proposals for revising the mix of clerical workers and radiography helpers, a new grade of associate radiographer, and fewer, but more highly trained, graduate radiographers (NHSME 1992; cited by Seccombe and Buchan 1994).

2 CONCEPTUALIZING THE NURSING ROLE

1 Irrespective of where their theories start from or the motors of change they predict most sociologists have held to the basic assumption that as societies develop, work becomes more complex and the division of labour more specialized. Dingwall, (1983b) has suggested that these assumptions may be overly simplistic. On the basis of an analysis of the development of

180

health visiting Dingwall suggests the addition of two further concepts: occupational fusion and occupational capture.

2 Hughes himself elides this distinction on occasion.

3 THE STUDY

1 Towards the end of my observations on Treetops, bed occupancy was unusually low as one of the urologists had reduced the number of his admissions dramatically because he was leaving the hospital. Moreover, fieldwork over-lapped with the pre Christmas period when routine operations were stopped, a further factor that influenced bed occupancy.

2 These figures do not add up because one person was interviewed more than once and two auxiliaries were interviewed together.

4 THE INTRA-OCCUPATIONAL DIVISION OF LABOUR

1 These findings are consistent with those of Mead and McGuire (1993) who found that only 3 per cent of the wards they surveyed were utilizing a primary nursing system.

5 THE NURSE–SUPPORT WORKER BOUNDARY

1 Wolf (1988) concludes that the symbolic meaning of post-mortem ritual rests in the nurses' need to remove the manifestations of suffering, to 'purify the patient's body and the hospital room of the soil and profanity of death, and to gradually relinquish their tenure of responsibility for the patient, given up only as the escort personnel transports the dead patient to the morgue.' (Wolf 1988: 139).

6 THE NURSE–MANAGEMENT BOUNDARY

1 Harrison and Pollitt (1994) note that 'quality' issues were divided up along tribal lines. Nurses had responsibility for Total Quality Management of the service, but the quality of medicine remained a medical affair.

2 The new public management in education has had a similar effect on teachers. See, for example Menter and Muschamp (1999) who report on the increased administrative burdens the introduction of a National Curriculum created for teachers.

3 Although care plans may be of little use to experienced nurses they are potentially of value to support staff. Nevertheless, at Woodlands care plans were not utilized by auxiliaries or HCAs who saw them as the province of qualified staff and of little relevance to them or their work.

4 Peters and Waterman's *In Search Of Excellence: Lessons from American's Best Run Companies,* seems to have acted as a catalyst for the development of the 'excellence' approach to management to rival the older management system whose components were Taylorism, Fordism and scientific management (Pfeffer and Coote 1991).

5 Griffiths and Hughes (2000) have also observed how other healthcare workers mediate management and professional discourses in the context of the contracting process.

6 This refers to NHSME (1993) *A Vision for the Future: Nursing, Midwifery and Health Visiting Contribution to Health and Health Care,* London: DH.

NOTES

7 THE NURSE–DOCTOR BOUNDARY

1 Similar arguments were made in the US in the 1970s. Nurses' initial resistance to the development of the nurse practitioner role was overcome in the face of the threat posed to them by the development of the non-nursing physician's assistant role.
2 A directorate is a unit of management within the Trust. In this hospital the medical and surgical services were separate directorates.
3 The Admissions Unit was created primarily with the needs of junior doctors in mind. The unit acted as a 'buffer' for medical emergencies admitted to the hospital. Patients could stay on the unit for up to 48 hours where their condition could be assessed, and if deemed necessary, an appropriate bed found on one of the wards. The Admissions Unit concentrated on the efficient processing and disposal of patients; it increased the efficiency of on-call doctors by concentrating all acute medical admissions in one area rather than placing them in different wards around the hospital.

9 CONCLUSIONS

1 Relatives were also being encouraged to involve themselves in ward work in response to the pressures of work on staff. Consider the following, for example: 'With a helpless patient, the ward Sister may welcome your offer to help during meal times. The patient may appreciate your personal help and it certainly can reduce the load on busy nurses.' (Document – *'Information for Visitors'*)
2 Although the model may be appropriate for nursing work in the community context it is a poor reflection of hospital-based care.

BIBLIOGRAPHY

Abbott, A. (1988) *The System of Professions: an Essay on the Division of Expert Labor*, Chicago: University of Chicago Press.

Aldridge, M. (1994) 'Unlimited liability? Emotional labour in nursing and social work', *Journal of Advanced Nursing* 20: 722–8.

Allen, D. (1996) 'The shape of general hospital nursing: the division of labour at work', PhD Thesis, University of Nottingham, UK.

— (1997a) 'The nursing–medical boundary: a negotiated order?', *Sociology of Health and Illness* 9(4): 498–520.

— (1997b) 'Nursing knowledge and practice', *Journal of Health Services Research and Policy* 2(3):190–4.

— (2000) 'Negotiating the role of 'expert carers' on an adult hospital ward', *Sociology of Health and Illness* 22(2): 149–71.

Allen, D. and Hughes, D. (1993) 'Going for growth', *Health Service Journal* 103(5372): 33–4.

Allen, D. and Lyne, P. (1997) 'Nurses' flexible working practices: some ethnographic insights into clinical effectiveness', *Clinical Effectiveness in Nursing* 1: 131–40.

Allen, D., Hughes, D. and Pickersgill, F. (1993) 'Receptivity to expanded nursing roles: the views of junior doctors, nurses and health care assistants', Paper presented at Nurse Practitioners: the UK/USA experience conference, The Cafe Royal, London.

Allsop, J. (1984) *Health Policy and the National Health Service*, London and New York: Longman.

— (1995) *Health Policy and the NHS: Towards 2000* (2nd edn), London: Longman.

Anderson, R. and Bury, M. (1988) *Living with Chronic Illness: the Experience of Patients and their Families*, London: Hyman Unwin.

Annandale, E. (1996) 'Working on the front-line: risk culture and nursing in the new NHS', *Sociological Review* 44(3): 416–51.

— (1998) *The Sociology of Health and Medicine: a Critical Introduction*, Cambridge: Polity.

Anspach, R.R. (1993) *Deciding Who Lives: Fateful Choices in the Intensive-Care Nursery*, Los Angeles: University of California Press.

Antaki, C. and Widdicombe, S. (eds) (1998) *Identities in Talk*, London: Sage.

Appleby, J., Walsh, K. and Ham, C. (1995) 'Acting on the evidence', Research paper, London National Association for Health Authorities and Trusts.

Apter, T. (1993) *Professional Progress: Why Women Still Don't Have Wives*, London: Macmillan Press.

Armstrong, D. (1983) 'The fabrication of nurse–patient relationships', *Social Science and Medicine* **17**(8): 457–60.

Atkinson, P. (1992) 'The ethnography of a medical setting: reading, writing, and rhetoric', *Qualitative Health Research* **2**(4): 451–74.

Baker, S. and Lyne, P. (1996) 'Quality and patients' expectations of a surgical admission', *Seminars in Pre-operative Nursing* **5**(4): 441–7.

Ball, J.A. and Goldstone, L.A. (1987) 'But who will make the beds? A report of the Mersey Region project on assessment of nurse staffing and support worker requirements for acute general hospitals', Merseyside Regional Health Authority: Nuffield Institute for Health Services Studies.

Barker, P.J., Reynolds, W. and Ward, T. (1995) 'The proper focus of nursing: a critique of the 'caring' ideology', *International Journal of Nursing Studies* **32**(4): 386–97.

Beardshaw, V. and Robinson, R. (1990) *New for Old? Prospects for Nursing in the 1990s*, London: Kings Fund Institute.

Becker, H.S. (1970) 'The nature of a profession', in H.S. Becker (ed.) *Sociological Work*, Chicago: Aldine.

Benner, P. (1984) *From Novice to Expert – Excellence and Power in Clinical Nursing Practice*, Menlo Park, CA: Addison and Wesley.

Benson, J.K. (1977a) 'Organizations: a dialectic view', *Administrative Science Quarterly* **22**: 1–21.

—— (1977b) 'Innovation and crisis in organizational analysis', *Sociological Quarterly* **18**: 5–18.

—— (1978) 'Reply to Maines', *Sociological Quarterly* **19**: 497–501.

Bergen, A. (1999) 'Nursing as caring revisited', in I. Norman and S. Cowley (eds) *The Changing Nature of Nursing in a Managerial Age*, Oxford: Blackwell Science.

Berger, P. and Luckman, T. (1967) *The Social Construction of Reality*, London: Allen Lane.

Black, N. (1998) 'Clinical governance: fine words or action?', *British Medical Journal* **316**(7127): 297. Available online: http://www.bmj.com/cgi/content/full/316/7127/297

Bosk, C.L. (1979) *Forgive and Remember: Managing Medical Mistakes*, Chicago: The University of Chicago Press.

Bowers, L. (1989) 'The significance of primary nursing', *Journal of Advanced Nursing* **14**: 13–19.

Bradley, H. (1989) *Men's Work, Women's Work: a Sociological History of the Sexual Division of Labour in Employment*, Minneapolis: University of Minnesota Press.

Brannon, R.L. (1994) *Intensifying Care: the Hospital Industry, Professionalization, and the Reorganization of the Nursing Labor Process*, New York: Baywood Publishing Company.

Brearley, S. (1990) *Patient Participation: the Literature*, London: Scutari.

Brown, J. (1990) 'Creating opportunities from challenges', Paper presented to the annual conference of the Royal College of Nursing.

Brownlea, A. (1987) 'Participation: myths, realities and prognosis', *Social Science and Medicine* 25(6): 605–14.

Buchan, J. (1992) 'Flexibility or fragmentation: trends and prospects in nurses' pay', Briefing Paper No 13, London: Kings Fund Institute.

Bucher, R. and Stelling, J. (1977) *Becoming Professional*, Beverly Hills: Sage.

Buckenham, J. and McGrath, G. (1983) *The Social Reality of Nursing*, Baglowalah, Australia: Adis Health Science Press.

Burgess, R.G. (1984) *In the Field: an Introduction to Field Research*, London and New York: Routledge.

Busch, L. (1982) 'History, negotiation and structure in agricultural research', *Urban Life* 11: 368–84.

Campbell, T. (1981) *Seven Theories of Human Society*, Oxford: Oxford University Press.

Carlin, B. and Mahony, C. (1999) 'Boss's pay-off an insult to nurses, says angry MP', *Nursing Times* 95(43): 9.

Carpenter, M. (1977) 'The new managerialism and professionalism in nursing', in M. Stacey, M. Reid, C. Heath and R. Dingwall (eds) *Health and the Division of Labour*, London: Croom Helm.

— (1978) 'Managerialism and the division of labour in nursing', in R. Dingwall and J. McIntosh (eds) *Readings in the Sociology of Nursing*, Edinburgh, London, New York: Churchill Livingstone.

— (1993) 'The subordination of nurses in health care: towards a social divisions approach', in E. Riska and K. Wegar (eds) *Gender Work and Medicine: Women and the Medical Division of Labour*, London: Sage.

Caress, A.L. (1997) 'Patient roles in decision-making', *Nursing Times* 93(31): 45–8.

Casey, N. (1995a) 'Editorial', *Nursing Standard* 9(19): 3.

— (1995b) 'Editorial', *Nursing Standard*, 9(43): 3.

Clarke, M. (1978) 'Getting through the work', in R. Dingwall and J. McIntosh (eds) *Readings in the Sociology of Nursing*, Edinburgh, London, New York: Churchill Livingstone.

Closs, S.J. and Cheater, F.M. (1999) 'Evidence for nursing practice: a clarification of the issues', *Journal of Advanced Nursing* 30(1): 10–17.

Cohan, M. (1997) 'Political identities and political landscapes: men's narrative work in relation to women's issues', *Sociological Quarterly* 38(2): 303–19.

Cook, J. (1994) 'The sacking of Sister Pat', *The Guardian*, (October 5th): 18.

Coombes, R. (2000) 'Nurses fearful of new times', *Nursing Times* 96(6): 4.

Corley, M. and Mauksch, H. (1988) 'Registered nurses, gender and commitment', in A. Stratham, E. Miller and H. Mauksch (eds) *The Worth of Women's Work: a Qualitative Synthesis*, New York: State University Press.

Crompton, R. and Sanderson, K. (1990) *Gendered Jobs and Social Change*, London: Unwin Hyman.

Darbyshire, P. (1994) *Living With a Sick Child in Hospital: the Experiences of Parents and Nurses*, London: Chapman and Hall.

Davies, C. (1977) 'Continuities in the development of hospital nursing in Britain', *Journal of Advanced Nursing* **1**(2): 479–93.

—— (1983) 'Professionalising strategies as time and culture bound: American and British Nursing 1983', in E. Condliffe Lagemann (ed.) *Nursing History: New Perspectives, New Possibilities*, New York: Teachers College Press.

—— (1995) *Gender and the Professional Predicament in Nursing*, Buckingham: Open University Press.

Davies, C. and Rosser, J. (1986) 'Gendered jobs in the health service: a problem for labour process analysis', in D. Knights and H. Willmott (eds) *Gender and the Labour Process*, Aldershot, Hampshire: Gower.

Davis, F. (1972) 'Uncertainty in medical prognosis, clinical and functional', in E. Freidson and J. Lorber (eds), *Medical Men and Their Work*, Chicago: Aldine, Atherton Inc.

Dawe, A. (1970) 'The two sociologies', *British Journal of Sociology* **21**: 207–18.

Day, R.A. and Day, J.V. (1977) 'A review of the current state of negotiated order theory: an appreciation and critique', *Sociological Quarterly* **18**: 126–42.

—— (1978) 'Reply to Maines', *Sociological Quarterly* **19**: 499–501.

De la Cuesta, C. (1983) 'The "Nursing Process" from development to implementation', *Journal of Advanced Nursing* **8**: 365–71.

Deal, T. and Kennedy, A. (1982) *Corporate Cultures: the Rites and Rituals of Corporate Life*, Cambridge, MA: Addison Wesley.

Deegan, M. (1995) 'The second sex and the Chicago School: women's accounts, knowledge, and work 1945–1960', in G. Fine (ed.) *A Second Chicago School? The Development of a Post War American Sociology*, Chicago: University of Chicago Press.

Dent, M. (1993) Professionalism, educated labour and the state – hospital medicine and the new managerialism', *Sociological Review* **41**: 244–73.

Dex, S. (1985) *The Sexual Division of Work: Conceptual Revolutions in the Social Sciences*, Sussex: Wheatsheaf Books Ltd.

Dey, I. (1993) *Qualitative Data Analysis*, London: Routledge.

DH (1989a) *Working for Patients: The Health Service Caring for the 1990s*, London: HMSO.

—— (1989b) *Working For Patients: Education and Training; Working Paper 10*, DH.

—— (1992) *The Health of the Nation: a Strategy for Health in England*, London: HMSO.

—— (1998a) *The New NHS Modern and Dependable: a National Framework for Assessing Performance*, London: HMSO. Available online: http://www.doh.gov.uk/newnhs/popular/pop2~1.htm.

—— (1998b) *Our Healthier Nation*, London: DH. Available online: http://www.official-documents.co.uk/document/doh/ohnation/title.htm.

—— (1998c) *Policy Research Programme: Health in Partnership Research Initiative*, London: DH.

— (1998d) *A First Class Service: Quality in the New NHS*, London: DH.

— (1999a) 'Biggest nursing pay rise for 10 years – paid in full', DH. wysiwyg:// Main.40/http://porch.ccta.gov.uk (February 1999).

— (1999b) *Improving Working Lives*, DH.

— (1999c) *Making a Difference: Strengthening the Nursing, Midwifery and Health Visiting Contribution to Health and Health Care*, DH. Available online: http://www.doh.gov.uk/nursrat.htm.

— (2000a) *The NHS Plan. A plan for investment. A plan for reform.* Cmnd 4818-I, Norwich, HMSO. Available online: www.nhs.uk/nhsplan

— (2000b) *A Health Service of all the Talents. Developing the NHS workforce.* Consultation document on the review of workforce planning, DH. Available online: www.doh.gov.uk/wfprconsult.

DHSS (1972) Report of the Committee on Nursing (Chairman, Lord Briggs), cmnd. 5115, London: HMSO.

— (1983) *Inquiry into NHS Management* (The Griffiths Report). London: DHSS.

— (1986) *Mix and Match: A Review of Nursing Skill Mix*, DHSS.

— (1987) *Hospital Medical Staffing (Achieving a Balance) – Plan for Action.* Health Circular, 87 (25), London: HMSO.

— (1995) *Health and Personal Social Services Statistics for England*, London: HMSO.

DHSS and Welsh Office (1979) *Patients First: Consultative Paper on the Structure and Management of the National Health Service in England and Wales*, London: HMSO.

DHSS, Northern Ireland (1998) *Fit for the Future*, Northern Ireland: DHSS.

Diamond, T. (1988) 'Social policy and everyday life in nursing homes: a critical ethnography', in A. Stratham, E. Miller and H. Mauksch (eds) *The Worth of Women's Work: a Qualitative Synthesis*, New York: State University Press.

Dickson, N. and Cole, A. (1987) 'Nurse's little helper?', *Nursing Times* **83**(10): 24–6.

Dingwall, R. (1977a) *The Social Organisation of Health Visitor Training*, London: Croom Helm.

— (1977b) 'Atrocity stories and professional relationships', *Sociology of Work and Occupations* **4**: 317–96.

— (1980) 'Ethics and ethnography', *Sociological Review* **28**(4): 871–91.

— (1983a) 'Introduction', in R. Dingwall and P. Lewis (eds) *The Sociology of the Professions: Lawyers, Doctors and Others*, London: Macmillan.

— (1983b) 'In the beginning was the work ... reflections on the genesis of occupations', *Sociological Review* **31**: 605–24.

Dingwall, R. and Strong, P. (1985) 'The interactional study of organization: a critique and reformulation', *Urban Life* **14**(2): 205–31.

Dingwall, R., Eekelaar, J. and Murray, T. (1983) *The Protection of Children: State Intervention and Family Life*, London: Basil Blackwell.

Dingwall, R., Rafferty, A.M. and Webster, C. (1988) *An Introduction to the Social History of Nursing*, London: Routledge.

Douglas, M. (1966) *Purity and Danger: an Analysis of Concepts of Pollution and Taboo*, London: Routledge and Kegan Paul.

DTI (1989) *Opening New Markets: New Policies on Restrictive Trade Practices*, Cmnd. 727, London: HMSO.

— (1999) 'Workers gain new protection from extension of working time directive', DTI. wysiwyg://Main.40/http://porch.ccta.gov.uk (May 1999).

Dunlop, M.J. (1986) 'Is a science of caring possible?', *Journal of Advanced Nursing* **11**: 661–70.

Durkheim, E. (1933) *The Division of Labour in Society*, London: Collier-Macmillan Ltd.

Eisenstein, Z.R. (1979) 'Developing a theory of capitalist patriarchy and socialist feminism', in Z.R. Eisenstein (ed.) *Capitalist Patriarchy*, New York: Monthly Review Press.

Elkan, R., Hillman, R. and Robinson, J. (1993) 'The implementation of Project 2000 in a District Health Authority: the effect on the nursing service', Nursing Policy Studies 10: Nottingham, University of Nottingham, Department of Nursing and Midwifery Studies.

— (1994) 'Project 2000 and the replacement of the traditional student workforce', *International Journal of Nursing Studies* **31**(5): 413–20.

Elston, M.A. (1991) 'The politics of professional power: medicine in a changing health service', in J. Gabe, M. Calnan and M. Bury (eds) *The Sociology of the Health Service*, London and New York: Routledge.

Emerson, R. and Pollner, M. (1976) 'Dirty work designations: their features and consequences in a psychiatric setting', *Social Problems* **23**: 243–54.

Ersser, S.J. (1997) *Nursing as a Therapeutic Activity: an Ethnography*, Aldershot: Avebury.

Etzioni, A. (1969) *The Semi-Professions and their Organization*, New York: Free Press.

Exworthy, M. (1998) 'Clinical audit in the NHS internal market: from peer review to external monitoring', *Public Policy and Administration* **13**: 40–53.

Fairhurst, E. (1977) 'On being a patient in an orthopaedic ward: some thoughts on the definition of the situation', in A. Davies and G. Horobin (eds) *Medical Encounters: the Experience of Illness and Treatment*, London: Croom Helm.

Finlay, W., Mutran, E.J., Zeitler, R.R. and Randall, C.S. (1990) 'Queues and care: how medical residents organise their work in a busy clinic', *Journal of Health and Social Behaviour* **31**: 292–305.

Flynn, N. (1990) *Public Sector Management*, Hemel Hempstead: Harvester Wheatsheaf.

FolioViews Infobase Production Kit version 3.1 (1995) Folio Corporation.

Foucault, M. (1976) *The Birth of the Clinic*, London: Tavistock.

Friend, J.K., Power, J.M., and Yewlett, C.J.L. (1974) *Public Planning: the Inter-Corporate Dimension*, London: Tavistock.

Freidson, E. (1970a) *Professional Dominance*, New York: Atherton Press Inc.

— (1970b) *Profession of Medicine: a Study in the Sociology of Applied Knowledge*, New York: Dodd, Mead and Co.

— (1976) 'The division of labour as social interaction', *Social Problems* **23**: 304–13.

— (1978) 'The official construction of work: an essay on the practical epistemology of occupations', Paper presented at the ninth World Congress of Sociology, Uppsala.

— (1983) 'The theory of professions: state of the art', in R. Dingwall and P. Lewis (eds) *The Sociology of the Professions: Lawyers, Doctors and Others*, London and Basingstoke: Macmillan Press.

Gamarnikow, E. (1978) 'Sexual division of labour; the case of nursing', in A. Kuhn and A.M. Wolpe (eds) *Feminism and Materialism: Women and Modes of Production*, London: Routledge and Kegan Paul.

— (1991) 'Nurse or woman: gender and professionalism in reformed nursing 1860–1923', in P. Holden and J. Littleworth (eds) *Anthropology and Nursing*, London: Routledge.

Garfinkel, H. (1967) *Studies in Ethnomethodology*, Engelwood Cliffs, NJ: Prentice Hall.

Geertz, C. (1983) *Local knowledge*, New York: Basic Books.

Giddens, A. (1979) *Central Problems in Social Theory: Action, Structure and Contradiction in Social Analysis*, London: Macmillan.

— (1984) *The Constitution of Society*, Cambridge: Polity Press.

Gieryn, T. (1983) '"Boundary-work" and the demarcation of science from non-science: strains and interests in professional ideologies of scientists', *American Sociological Review* **48**: 781–95.

— (1999) *Cultural Boundaries of Science: Credibility on the Line*, Chicago and London: The University of Chicago Press.

Glaser, B. and Strauss, A.L. (1965) *Awareness of Dying*, Chicago: Aldine Publishing Company.

— (1968) *Time for Dying*, Chicago: Aldine.

Glazer, N. (1993) *Women's Paid and Unpaid Labor: the Work Transfer in Health Care and Retailing*, Philadelphia: Templeton University Press.

GMC (1993) *Tomorrow's Doctors.* London: GMC.

GNC (1977) *A Statement of Educational Policy*, July 1977, circular 77/19/A.

Goddard, H.A. (1953) *The Work of Nurses in Hospital Wards*, Nuffield Provincial Hospital Trust.

Goffman, E. (1959) *The Presentation of Self in Everyday Life*, Harmondsworth: Penguin Books Ltd.

— (1961) *Asylums: Essays on the Social Situation of Mental Patients and Other Inmates*, Harmondsworth: Penguin Books.

Gould, K. (1988) 'Old wine in new bottles: a feminist perspective on Gilligan's theory', *Social Work* **33**(5): 411–15.

Griffiths, L. and Hughes, D. (2000) 'Talking contracts and talking care: managers and professionals in the NHS internal market', *Social Science and Medicine* **51**: 209–22.

Gubrium, J. (1988) *Analyzing Field Realities*, Beverly Hills, CA: Sage.

— (1989) 'Local cultures and service policy', in J.F. Gubrium and D. Silverman (eds) *The Politics of Field Research*, London: Sage.

Gubrium, J.F. and Buckholdt, D.R. (1979) 'Production of hard data in human service institutions', *Pacific Sociological Review* **22**(1): 115–36.

Haas, J. and Shaffir, W. (1987) *Becoming Doctors: the Adoption of the Cloak of Competence*, London: JAI Press.

Hafferty, F.W. (1988) 'Cadaver stories and the emotional socialization of medical students', *Journal of Health and Social Behaviour* **29**: 344–56.

Hall, P.M. and Spencer-Hall, D.A. (1982) 'The social conditions of the negotiated order', *Urban Life* **11**: 328–49.

Ham, C. (1992) *Health Policy in Britain*, London: Macmillan Press.

Hakim, C. (1979) *Occupational Segregation: a Comparative Study of the Degree and Pattern of the Differentiation Between Men and Women's Work in Britain, the United States and Other Countries*, London: Department of Employment.

Hammersley, M. and Atkinson, P. (1983) *Ethnography: Principles in Practice*, London and New York: Routledge.

Hargreaves, A. (1981) 'Contrastive rhetoric and extremist talk' in P. Woods (ed.) *Schools, Teachers and Teaching*, Milton Keynes, UK: Open University Press.

Harrison, A. and Bruscini, S. (eds) (1995) *Health Care UK 1994/5*, London: Kings Fund Policy Institute.

Harrison, S. and Pollitt, C. (1994) *Controlling Health Professionals*, Milton Keynes, UK: Open University Press.

Harrison, S., Hunter, D.J. and Pollit, C. (1990) *The Dynamics of British Health Policy*, London: Unwin Hyman.

Hart, E. (1989) 'A qualitative study of micro level factors affecting staff retention and turnover amongst nursing staff in paediatrics and care of the elderly', A research report for Miss Hazel Miller, Regional Nursing Officer, Trent Regional Health Authority, Nottingham: Department of Nursing Studies, Queens Medical School.

Hartmann, H. (1979) 'The unhappy marriage of Marxism and feminism: towards a more progressive union', *Capital and Class* **8**: 1–33.

— (1981) 'The unhappy marriage of feminism and Marxism: towards a more progressive union', in L. Sargent (ed.) *Women and Revolution: the Unhappy Marriage of Marxism and Feminism*, London: Pluto Press.

Harvey-Jones, J. (1989) *Making it Happen: Reflections on Leadership*, Glasgow: Fontana/Collins.

Heimer, C.A. (1998) 'The routinization of responsiveness: regulatory compliance and the construction of organizational routines', American Bar Foundation working paper: 9801.

Hendry, J. and Martinez, L. (1991) 'Nursing in Japan', in P. Holden and J. Littlewood (eds) *Anthropology and Nursing*, London and New York: Routledge.

Heritage, J. (1984) *Garfinkel and Ethnomethodology*, Oxford: Polity Press.

Hochschild, A.R. (1983) *The Managed Heart: Commercialization of Human Feeling*, Berkeley: University of California Press.

— (1990) *The Second Shift: Working Parents and the Revolution at Home*, London: Judy Piatkus.

Hoggett, P. (1996) 'New modes of control in the public service', *Public Administration*, **74**: 9–32.

Homans, H. (1987) 'Man-made myths: the reality of being a woman scientist in the NHS', in A. Spencer and D. Podmore (eds) *In a Man's World*, London: Tavistock Publications.

Hood, C. (1991) 'A public management for all seasons', *Public Administration* **69**(1): 3–19.

Horton, R. (1997) 'Health a complicated game of doctors and nurses', *The Observer* 30 March.

Hughes, D. (1988) 'When nurse knows best: some aspects of nurse–doctor interaction in a casualty department', *Sociology of Health and Illness* **10**: 1–22.

Hughes, D. and Allen, D. (1993a) 'Inside the black box: obstacles to change in the modern hospital', Kings Fund and Milbank Memorial Fund: Joint Health Policy Review: School of Sociology and Social Policy, University of Nottingham.

— (1993b) 'Expanded nursing roles, junior doctors' hours and the hospital division of labour: a pilot study', South East Thames Regional Health Authority.

Hughes, D. and Griffiths, L. (1999) 'On penalties and the Patient's charter: centralism vs de-centralised governance in the NHS', *Sociology of Health and Illness* **21**(1): 71–94.

Hughes, E.C. (1984) *The Sociological Eye*, New Brunswick and London: Transaction Books.

Hughes, E.C., Hughes, H. and Deutscher, I. (1958) *Twenty Thousand Nurses Tell Their Story*, Philadelphia: JB Lippincott.

Hughes, P. (1993) 'The implications of NVQs for nursing', *Nursing Standard* **19**: 29.

Humphreys, J. (1996) 'English nurse education and the reform of the National Health Service', *Journal of Education Policy* **11**: 655–79.

Hunt, S.A. and Benford, R.D. (1994) 'Identity talk in the peace and justice movement', *Journal of Contemporary Ethnography* **22**(4): 488–517.

Hunter, D. (1990) '"Managing the cracks": management development for health care interfaces', *International Journal of Health Planning and Management* **5**: 7–14.

— (1998) 'The new health policy agenda: the challenge facing managers and researchers', *Research Policy and Planning* **16**(2): 2–7.

HSMU (1996) 'The future health care workforce: the steering group report', Health Services Management Unit: University of Manchester.

Illich, I. (1976) *Medical Nemesis: the Expropriation of Health*, London: Marion Boyars.

James, N. (1989) 'Emotional labour: skill and work in the social regulation of feelings', *Sociological Review* **37**: 15–41.

— (1992a) 'Care, work and carework: a synthesis?', in J. Robinson, A. Gray and R. Elkan (eds) *Policy Issues in Nursing*, Milton Keynes, UK: Open University Press.

— (1992b) 'Care = organisation + physical labour + emotional labour', *Sociology of Health and Illness* **14**(4): 488–509.

Jamous, H. and Peloille, B. (1970) 'Changes in the French university-hospital system', in J.A. Jackson (ed.) *Professions and Professionalization*, Cambridge: Cambridge University Press.

Johnson, J.M. (1975) *Doing Field Research*, London: Macmillan.

Johnson, T.J. (1967) *Professions and Power*, London: Macmillan.

Kelly, M. and May, D. (1982) 'Good and bad patients: a review of the literature and a theoretical critique', *Journal of Advanced Nursing* 7: 147–56.

Keyzer, D.M. (1988) 'Challenging role boundaries: conceptual frameworks for understanding the conflict arising from the implementation of the nursing process in practice', in R. White (ed.) *Political Issues in Nursing: Past, Present and Future*, London and New York: John Wiley and Sons.

Klein, R. (1995) *The New Politics of the NHS* (3rd edn), London and New York: Longman.

— (1997) 'The Kings Fund and the future of health policy', *Kings Fund News* **20**(1): 8–9.

Kleinman, S. (1982) 'Actors' conflicting theories of negotiation: the case of an holistic health center', *Urban Life* **11**(3): 312–27.

Lambert, C. (1999) 'In the red', *Nursing Times* **95**(43): 16.

Larson, M.S. (1977) *The Rise of Professionalism: a Sociological Analysis*, Berkeley: University of California Press.

Lawler, J. (1991) *Behind the Screens: Nursing, Somology and the Problem of the Body*, London: Churchill Livingstone.

Lawson, N. (1996) 'Is it the end nurses?', *The Times* Thursday 26 December.

Levy, J.A. (1982) 'The staging of negotiations between hospice and medical institutions', *Urban Life* **11**(3): 293–311.

Lipley, N. (1999) 'NHS ombudsman warns nurse shortages are leading relatives to make more complaints', *Nursing Standard* **13**(40): 4–5.

Lipsky, M. (1980) *Street-Level Bureaucracy: Dilemmas of the Individual in Public Services*, New York: Russell Sage Publications.

Littlewood, J. (1991) 'Care and ambiguity: towards a concept of nursing', in P. Holden and J. Littlewood (eds) *Anthropology and Nursing*, London: Routledge.

Loudon, J.B. (1977) 'On body products', in J. Blacking (ed.) *The Anthropology of the Body*, London, Academic Press.

Lyne, P. (1998) 'The future of nursing, midwifery and health visiting', NHSC Report 1, Nursing, Health and Social Care Research Centre, School of Nursing and Midwifery Studies, University of Wales College of Medicine, Cardiff.

Macintyre, S. and Oldman, D. (1977) 'Coping with migraine', in A. Davis and G. Horobin (eds) *Medical Encounters: the Experience of Illness and Treatment*, London: Croom Helm.

MacPherson, K.I. (1991) 'Looking at caring and nursing through a feminist lens', in R.M. Neil and R. Watts (eds) *Caring and Nursing: Explorations in Feminist Perspectives*, New York: National League for Nursing.

Mahony, C. (2000) 'The spin on nurses' hard work', *Nursing Times* **96**(10): 10.

Maines, D. (1977) 'Social organization and social structure in symbolic interactionist thought', *Annual Review of Sociology* **3**: 235–59.

—— (1982) 'In search of mesostructure: studies in the negotiated order', *Urban Life* **11**: 278–9.

Manthey, M. (1989) 'Practice partnerships: the newest concept in care delivery', *Journal of Nursing Administration* **19**(2): 33–5.

Mauksch, H.O. (1966), 'The organizational context of nursing practice', in F. Davis (ed.) *The Nursing Profession: Five Sociological Essays*, New York: John Wiley and Sons.

May, C. (1992) 'Nursing work, nurses' knowledge, and the subjectification of the patient', *Sociology of Health and Illness* **14**(4): 472–87.

May, D. and Kelly, M.P. (1982) 'Chancers, pests and poor wee souls: problems of legitimation in psychiatric nursing', *Sociology of Health and Illness* **4**(3): 279–97.

McFarlane, J.K. (1976) 'A charter for caring', *Journal of Advanced Nursing* **1**: 187–96.

McIntosh, J. (1977) *Communication and Awareness in a Cancer Ward*, London: Croom Helm.

McKee, M. and Lessof, L. (1992) 'Nurse and doctor: whose task is it anyway?', in J. Robinson, A. Gray, and R. Elkan (eds) *Policy Issues in Nursing*, Milton Keynes, UK: Open University Press.

McBarnet, D. and Whelan, C. (1991) 'The elusive spirit of the law: formalism and the struggle for legal control', *Modern Law Review*, **54**(6): 874–88.

McKenna, H., Cutcliffe, J. and McKenna, P. (2000) 'Evidence-based practice: demolishing some myths', *Nursing Standard* **14**(16): 39–41.

McKeown, T. (1965) *Medicine in Modern Society*, London: George Allen and Unwin.

McKibbon, K.A. and Walker, C.J. (1994) 'Beyond ACP journal club: how to harness Medline for therapy problems', *Annals of Internal Medicine* **121**(1): 125–7.

Mead, D. and McGuire, J. (1993) *Innovations in Nursing Practice: the Development of Primary Nursing in Wales*, NHS Wales.

Mechanic, D. (1961) 'Sources of power of lower participants in complex organisations', *Administrative Science Quarterly* **7**: 349–64.

Meerabeau, L. (1992) 'Tacit knowledge: an untapped resource or a methodological headache?', *Journal of Advanced Nursing* **17**: 108–12.

—— (1998) 'Project 2000 and the nature of nursing knowledge', in P. Abbott and L. Meerabeau (eds) *The Sociology of the Caring Professions* (2nd edn), London: UCL Press.

Melia, K. (1979) 'A sociological approach to the analysis of nursing work', *Journal of Advanced Nursing* **4**: 57–67.

—— (1987) *Learning and Working: the Occupational Socialization of Nurses*, London: Tavistock.

Mellinger, W.M. (1994) 'Negotiated orders: the negotiation of directives in paramedic-nurse interaction', *Symbolic Interaction* **17**: 165–85.

Menter, I. and Muschamp, Y. (1999) 'Markets and management: the case of primary schools', in M. Exworthy and S. Halford (eds) *Professionals and the New Managerialism in the Public Sector*, Milton Keynes, UK: Open University Press.

Menzies, I. (1963) 'A case study in the functioning of social systems as a defence against anxiety: a report on a study of the nursing service of a general hospital', *Human Relations* **13**: 95–121.

Miles, M.B. and Huberman, A.M. (1994) *Qualitative Data Analysis: an Expanded Source Book* (2nd edn), Thousand Oaks, CA: Sage.

Miller, G. (1997) 'Towards ethnographies of institutional discourse: proposals and suggestions', in G. Miller and R. Dingwall (eds) *Context and Method in Qualitative Research*, London: Sage.

Miller, G. and Holstein, J.A. (1993) 'Disputing in organizations: dispute domains and interactional process', *Mid-American Review of Sociology* **17**(2): 1–18.

Mills, C.W. (1940) 'Situated action and vocabularies of motive', in J.G. Manis and B.N. Meltzer (eds) *Symbolic Interaction: a Reader in Social Psychology*, Boston: Allyn and Bacon.

Milne, D. (1985) '"The more things change the more they stay the same": factors affecting the implementation of the nursing process', *Journal of Advanced Nursing* **10**: 39–45.

Ministry of Health and Scottish Home and Health Department (1966) *Report of the Committee on Senior Nursing Staff Structure* (Chairman, B. Salmon), London: HMSO.

Moore, W.E. (1963) *Man, Time and Society*, New York and London: John Wiley and Sons.

Morrison, K. and Cowley, S. (1999) 'Idealised caring: the heart of nursing', in I. Norman and S. Cowley (eds) *The Changing Nature of Nursing in a Managerial Age*, Oxford: Blackwell Science.

Mumford, E. (1970) *Interns: From Students to Physicians*, Cambridge, MA: Harvard University Press.

Murcott, A. (1981) 'On the typification of "bad patients"', in P. Atkinson and C. Heath (eds) *Medical Work: Realities and Routines*, Farnborough, Hants: Gower.

Murphy, E. (1999) '"Breast is best": infant feeding decisions and maternal deviance', *Sociology of Health and Illness* **21**(2): 187–208.

Myers, L.C. (1979) *The Socialization of Neophyte Nurses*, MI: UMI Research Press.

Naish, J. (1990) 'Vision or nightmare?', *Nursing Standard*, **12**: 18-19.

— (1993) 'Power, politics and peril', in B. Dolan (ed.) *Project 2000: Reflection and Celebration*, London: Scutari Press.

Needleman, R. and Nelson, A. (1988) 'Policy implications: the worth of women's work', in A. Stratham, E. Miller and H. Mauksch (eds) *The Worth of Women's Work: a Qualitative Synthesis*, New York: State University New York.

Newman, M. (1986) *Health as Expanding Consciousness*, St Louis, MO: Mosby.

NHS Confederation (2000) 'The changing relationship between doctors and managers', Position paper submitted to Phase Two of the Bristol Royal Infirmary Inquiry.

NHS Wales (1998) *Putting Patients First*, London: HMSO.

NHSME (1991) *Junior Doctors: the New Deal*, London: NHSME.

NHSME (1992) *NHS Trusts: the First Twelve Months*, NHSME, London.

NHSME (1993) *A Vision for the Future: the Nursing, Midwifery and Health Visiting Contribution to Health and Health Care*, London: DH.

Nursing Times (1999) 'Californian skill-mix law revives calls for UK minimums', *Nursing Times* **95**(43): 7.

Oakley, A. (1974a) *Housewife*, London: Penguin Books.

— (1974b) *The Sociology of Housework*, Oxford: Martin Robertson.

— (1979) *From Here to Maternity: Becoming a Mother*, Harmondsworth: Penguin Books.

— (1984) 'The importance of being a nurse', *Nursing Times* **80**(50): 24–7.

Ouchi, W.G. (1981) *Theory Z: How American Businesses can Meet the Japanese Challenge*, Reading, MA.: Addison Wesley.

Packwood, T., Keen, J. and Buxton, M. (1991) *Hospitals in Transition: the Resource Management Experiment*, Milton Keynes, UK: Open University Press.

Parker, J., Gardner, G. and Wiltshire, J. (1992) 'Handover: the collective narrative of nursing practice', *Australian Journal of Advanced Nursing* **9**(3): 31–7.

Parse, R.R. (1981) *Man-Living-Health: a Theory of Nursing*, New York: Wiley.

Parsons, T. (1951) *The Social System*, London: Routledge and Kegan Paul.

Paton, C. (1993) 'Devolution and centralism in the National Health Service', *Social Policy and Administration* **27**(2): 83–108.

Pearson, A. (ed.) (1988) *Primary Nursing: Nursing in the Burford and Oxford Nursing Development Units*, London: Chapman and Hall.

Perry, A. (1993) 'A sociologists' view: the handmaiden's theory', in M. Jolley and G. Brykcynska (eds) *Nursing: its Hidden Agendas*, London: Edward Arnold.

Peters, T.J. (1987) *Thriving on Chaos: Handbook for a Management Revolution*, New York: Knopf: Distributed by Random House.

Peters, T.J and Waterman, R.H. (1982) *In Search of Excellence: Lessons From America's Best-run Companies*, New York: Harper and Row.

Pettigrew, A., McKee, L. and Ferlie, E. (1988) 'Understanding change in the NHS', *Public Administration* **66**: 297–317.

Pfeffer, N. and Coote, A. (1991) *Is Quality Good for You?: a Critical Review of Quality Assurance in Welfare Services*, London: Institute for Public Policy Research.

Phelan, M.P. and Hunt, S.A. (1998) 'Prison gang members' tattoos as identity work: the visual communication of moral careers', *Symbolic Interaction* **21**(3): 277–98.

Phillips, A. and Taylor, B. (1980) 'Sex and skill: notes towards a feminist economics', *Feminist Review* **6**: 79–88.

Pollitt, C. (1995) 'Justification by works or by faith? Evaluating the new public management', *Evaluation* **1**(2): 133–54.

Porter, S. (1991) 'A participant observation study of power relations between nurses and doctors in a general hospital', *Journal of Advanced Nursing* **16**: 728–35.

— (1992) 'The poverty of professionalization: a critical analysis of strategies for the occupational advancement of nursing', *Journal of Advanced Nursing* **17**: 720–6.

— (1995) *Nursing's Relationship with Medicine: a Critical Realist Ethnography.* Aldershot: Avesbury.

Power, M. (1999) *The Audit Society: Rituals of Verification*, Oxford: Oxford University Press.

Pringle, R. (1989) *Secretaries Talk: Sexuality, Power and Work*, London: Verso.

Proctor, S. (1989) 'The functioning of nursing routines in the management of a transient work force', *Journal of Advanced Nursing* **14**: 180–9.

Quint, J.C. (1972) 'Institutionalised practices of information control', in E. Freidson and J. Lorber (eds) *Medical Men and Their Work*, Chicago: Aldine, Atherton.

Rafferty, A.M. (1992) 'Nursing policy and the nationalization of nursing: the representation of 'crisis' and the 'crisis' of representation', in J. Robinson, A. Gray and R. Elkan (eds) *Policy Issues in Nursing*, Milton Keynes, UK: Open University Press.

— (1996) *The Politics of Nursing Knowledge*, London: Routledge.

Ranade, W. (1994) *A Future for the NHS? Health Care in the 1990s*, London and New York: Longman.

RCN (1985) *The Education of Nurses: a New Dispensation*, London: RCN.

Robertson, L. (ed.) (1994) *The Health Services Year Book 1994*, London: Institute of Health Services Management.

Robinson, J. (1992) 'Introduction: beginning the study of nursing policy', in J. Robinson, A. Gray and R. Elkan (eds) *Policy Issues in Nursing*, Milton Keynes, UK: Open University Press.

Robinson, J., Stilwell, J., Hawley, C. and Hempstead, N. (1989) 'The role of the support worker in the ward health care team', Nursing Policy Studies 6, Warwick: Nursing Policy Studies Centre, University of Warwick.

Robinson, R. (1994) 'Introduction', in R. Robinson and J. Le Grand (eds) *Evaluating the NHS Reforms*, Berks: Policy Journals.

Robinson, R. and Le Grand, J. (eds) (1994) Evaluating the NHS Reforms, Berks: Policy Journals.

Rosenfeld, D. (1999) 'Identity work among lesbian and gay elderly', *Journal of Aging Studies* **13**(2): 121–44.

Rosenthal, C., Marshall, V.W. and French, S.E. (1980) *Nurses, Patients and Families*, London: Croom Helm.

Roth, J.A. (1963) *Timetables: Structuring the Passage of Time in Hospital Treatment and Other Careers*, New York: The Bobbs-Merrill Company Inc.

— (1974) 'Professionalism: the sociologist's decoy', *Sociology of Work and Occupations* **1**: 6–23.

Roth, J. and Douglas, D. (1983) *No Appointment Necessary: the Hospital Emergency Department in the Medical Services World*, New York: Irving Publishers.

Rothman, B.K. and Detlefs, M. (1988) 'Women talking to women: abortion counsellors and genetic counsellors', in A. Stratham, E. Miller and H. Mauksch (eds) *The Worth of Women's Work: a Qualitative Synthesis*, New York: State University New York Press.

Salvage, J. (1985) *The Politics of Nursing*, London: Heinemann Nursing.

— (1988) 'Partnerships in care? An exploration of the theory and practice of the new nursing in the UK', MSc Thesis, Royal Holloway and Bedford New College, University of London.

— (1992) 'The New Nursing: empowering patients or empowering nurses?', in J. Robinson, A. Gray and R. Elkan (eds) *Policy Issues in Nursing*, Milton Keynes, UK: Open University Press.

— (1995) 'Political implications of the named-nurse concept', *Nursing Times* **91**(41): 36–7.

Samarel, N. (1991) *Caring for Life and Death*, London: Hemisphere Publishing Corporation.

Savage, J. (1987) *Nurses, Gender and Sexuality*, London: Heinemann Nursing.

— (1995) *Nursing Intimacy: an Ethnographic Approach to Nurse–Patient Interaction*, London: Scutari Press.

Sayer, A. (1996) 'Contractualisation, work and the anxious classes', Paper presented to the Swedish Council for Work Life Research Conference, 'Work Quo Vadis', University of Karlstad.

Scheff, T.J. (1961) 'Control over policy by attendants in a mental hospital', *Journal of Health and Human Behaviour* **2**: 93–105.

Schein, E.H. (1985) *Organisational Culture and Leadership: a Dynamic View*, San Francisco: Jossey-Bass.

Schön, D. (1971) *Beyond the Stable State*, London: Temple Smith.

Scott, M. and Lyman, S. (1968) 'Accounts', *American Sociological Review* **33**: 46–62

Scottish Office and Department of Health (1997) *Designed to Care: Renewing the National Health Service in Scotland*, Edinburgh: Scottish Office.

Seccombe, I. and Buchan, J. (1994) 'The changing role of the NHS personnel function', in R. Robinson. and J. Le Grand (eds) *Evaluating the NHS Reforms*, Berks: Policy Journals.

Shaw, I. (1993) 'The politics of inter-professional training – lessons from learning disability', *Journal of Inter-professional Care* **7**(3): 255–62.

Shotter, J. (1993) *Conversational Realities: Constructing Life Through Language*, London: Sage.

Silverman, D. (1993) *Interpreting Qualitative Data: Methods for Analysing Talk, Text and Interaction*, London: Sage.

Simmel, G. (1950) 'Superordination and subordination', in K.H. Wolf (ed.) *The Sociology of Georg Simmel*, New York: Free Press.

Smith, P. (1992) *The Emotional Labour of Nursing: How Nurses Care*, London: Macmillan Education.

Snow, D.A. and Anderson, L. (1987) 'Identity work among the homeless: the verbal construction and avowal of personal identities', *American Journal of Sociology* **92**(6): 1336–71.

Somjee, G. (1991) 'Social change in the nursing profession in India', in P. Holden and J. Littlewood (eds) *Anthropology in Nursing*, London: Routledge.

Stacey, M. (1976) 'The health service consumer: a sociological misconception', in M. Stacey (ed.) *The Sociology of the NHS*, Monograph 22, Stoke-on-Trent: Wood Mitchell and Co.

— (1981) 'The division of labour revisited or overcoming the two Adams', in P. Abrams, R. Deem, J. Finch and P. Rock (eds) *Practice and Progress: British Sociology 1950–1980*, London: George Allen and Unwin.

— (1992) *Regulating British Medicine: The General Medical Council*, Chichester: Wiley.

Stearns, C.A. (1991) 'Physicians in restraints: HMO gatekeepers and their perceptions of demanding patients', *Qualitative Health Research* **1**(3): 326–48.

Stein, L. (1967) 'The doctor–nurse game', *Archives of General Psychiatry* **16**: 699–703.

Stein, L., Watts, D.T. and Howell, T. (1990) 'The doctor–nurse game revisited', *Nursing Outlook* **36**: 264–8.

Strangleman, T. and Roberts, I. (1999) 'Looking through the window of opportunity: the cultural cleansing of workplace identity', *Sociology* **33**(1): 47–67.

Strauss, A.L. (1978) *Negotiations: Varieties, Contexts, Processes and Social Order*, London: Jossey-Bass.

— (1982) 'Social worlds and their segmentation processes', *Studies in Symbolic Interaction* **5**: 123–39.

Strauss, A., Schatzman, L., Bucher, R., Ehrlich, D. and Sabshin, M. (1963) 'The hospital and its negotiated order', in E. Freidson (ed.) *The Hospital in Modern Society*, New York: Free Press.

— (1964) *Psychiatric Ideologies and Institutions*, London: The Free Press of Glencoe Collier-Macmillan.

Strauss, A., Fagerhaugh, S., Suczet. B. and Wiener, C. (1985) *The Social Organisation of Medical Work*, Chicago: University of Chicago Press.

Strong, P. and Robinson, J. (1990) *The NHS Under New Management*, Milton Keynes, UK: Open University Press.

Sugrue, N.M. (1982) 'Emotions as property and context for negotiation', *Urban Life* **11**(3): 280–92.

Sutton, F. and Smith, C. (1995) 'Advanced nursing practice: new ideas and new perspectives', *Journal of Advanced Nursing* **21**: 1037–43.

Svensson, R. (1996) 'The interplay between doctors and nurses – a negotiated order perspective', *Sociology of Health and Illness* **18**(3): 379–98.

Titchen, A. and Binnie, A. (1993) 'What am I meant to be doing? Putting practice into theory and back again in new nursing roles', *Journal of Advanced Nursing* **18**: 1054–65.

Tomich, J.H. (1978) 'The expanded role of the nurse: current status and future prospects', in N. Chaska (ed.) *The Nursing Profession: Views Through the Mist*, New York: McGraw-Hill.

Towell, D. (1975) *Understanding Psychiatric Nursing*, London: Royal College of Nursing.

Travelbee, J. (1966) *Interpersonal Aspects of Nursing*, Philadelphia: FA Davis.

Traynor, M. (1999) *Managerialism and Nursing*, London: Routledge.

Trnobranski, P. (1994) 'Nurse–patient negotiation: assumption or reality?', *Journal of Advanced Nursing* **19**: 733–7.

Turner, B.S. (1986) 'The vocabulary of complaints: nursing, professionalism and job context', *ANZJS* **22**: 368–86.

UKCC (1987) *Project 2000: the Final Proposals*, London: UKCC.

— (1992) *The Scope of Professional Practice*, London: UKCC.

— (1999a) *A Higher Level of Practice: Draft Descriptor and Standard*, UKCC.

— (1999b) *A Higher Level of Practice: the UKCC's Proposals for Recognising a Higher Level of Practice within the Post Registration Regulatory Framework*, UKCC. Available online: http://www.ukcc.org.uk/ A%20higher%20level%of%20practice.htm.

— (1999c) *Fitness for Practice: the UKCC Commission for Nursing and Midwifery Education*, UKCC. Available online: http://www.ukcc.org.uk.

Ungerson, C. (1983) 'Women and caring: skills, tasks and taboos', in E. Gamarnikow, D. Morgan, J. Purvis and D. Taylorson (eds) *The Public and the Private*, London: Heinemann.

Walby, S. (1986) *Patriarchy at Work: Patriarchal and Capitalist Relations in Employment*, Cambridge: Polity Press.

— (1989) 'Flexibility and the changing sexual division of labour', in S. Woods (ed.) *The Transformation of Work*, London: Unwin Hyman.

Walby, S. and Greenwell, J. with MacKay, L. and Soothill, K. (1994) *Medicine and Nursing: Professions in a Changing Health Service*, London: Sage.

Walton, I. (1986) 'The nursing process in perspective: a literature review', University of York, Department of Social Policy and Social Work.

Watson, J. (1985) *Nursing: the Philosophy and Science of Caring*, Colorado: University Press of Colorado.

Wax, R. (1971) *Doing Fieldwork*, Chicago: University of Chicago Press.

Webb, C. and Pontin, D. (1996) 'Introducing primary nursing: nurses' opinions', *Journal of Clinical Nursing* **5**: 351–8.

Webb, J. (1999) 'Work and the new public service class?', *Sociology* **33**(4): 747–66.

Weber, M. (1970) *From Max Weber: Essays in Sociology*, London: Routledge and Kegan Paul.

Welsh Office and NHS Cymru Wales (1998) *NHS Wales: Putting Patients First*, WO.

White, R. (1986) 'From matron to manager: the political construction of reality', in R. White (ed.) *Political Issues in Nursing: Past, Present and Future*, New York and London: John Wiley and Sons.

Whyte, W.F. (1979) 'The social structure of the restaurant', in H. Robboy, S.L. Greenblatt and C. Clark (eds) *Social Interaction: Introductory Readings in Sociology*, New York: St Martin's Press.

Wicks, D. (1998) *Nurses and Doctors at Work: Rethinking Professional Boundaries*, Buckingham: Open University Press.

Williams, C. (2000) 'Alert assistants in managing chronic illness: the case of mothers and teenage sons', *Sociology of Health and Illness* **22**(2): 254–72.

Williams, G. and Popay, J. (1994) 'Lay knowledge and the privilege of experience', in J. Gabe, D. Kelleher and G. Williams (eds) *Challenging Medicine*, London: Routledge.

Willmott, M. (1998) 'The new ward manager: an evaluation of the changing role of the charge nurse', *Journal of Advanced Nursing* **28**(2): 419–27.

Witz, A. (1986) 'Patriarchy and the labour market: occupational control strategies and the medical division of labour', in D. Knights and H. Willmott (eds) *Gender and the Labour Process*, Hampshire: Gower.

—— (1988) 'Patriarchal relations and patterns of sex segregation in the medical division of labour', in S. Walby (ed.) *Gender Segregation at Work*, Milton Keynes, UK: Open University Press.

—— (1992) *Professions and Patriarchy*, London: Routledge.

—— (1994) 'The challenge of nursing' in J. Gabe, D. Kelleher and G. Williams (eds) *Challenging Medicine*, London: Routledge.

Wolf, Z.R. (1988) *Nurses' Work: The Sacred and the Profane*, Philadelphia: University of Pennsylvania Press.

—— (2000) 'Nursing rituals: doing ethnography', in P.L. Munhall and C.O. Boyd (eds) *Nursing Research: a Qualitative Perspective* (2nd edn) Sudbury, USA: Jones and Bartlett Publishers, National League for Nursing.

Wright, S. (1995) 'The role of the nurse: extended or expanded?', *Nursing Standard* **9**(33): 25–9.

Zerubavel, E. (1979) *Patterns of Time in Hospital Life*, Chicago: Chicago University Press.

INDEX